STRONG PEGAN MEAL FOR DINNER

FIND AND COOK YOUR BEST PROTEIN DINNER!

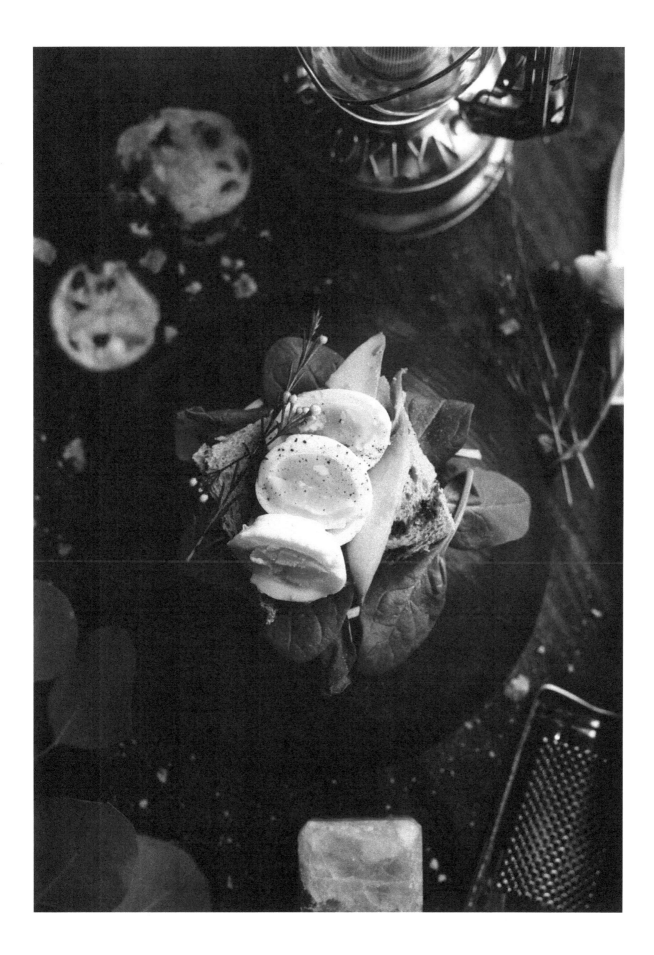

Table of Contents

Introduction

Chapter 1.   **What is the Pegan Diet?**

Chapter 2.   **Vegan Diet and Workout: Benefits and Disadvantages**

Chapter 3.   **Paleo Diet and Workout: Benefits and Disadvantages**

Chapter 4.   **The Importance of Nutrients: Where Do Vegans and Paleos Get Proteins, Fat, Carbs, Sugar and Fibers**

Chapter 5.   **What can a Pegan eat and What Cannot?**

Chapter 6.   **Protein Dinner**

1. *Belgian Endive Frittata*

2. *Carrot Frittata*

3. *Kale Frittata*

4. *Ham Frittata*

5. *Broccoli Frittata*

6. *Apple Slaw*

7. *Ground Beef with Peas*

8. *Beef with Lentils*

9. *Beef with Cauliflower*

10. *Glazed Flank Steak*

11. *Stuffed Turkey Breast*

12. *Grilled Chicken Breast*

13. *Glazed Chicken Thighs*

14. *Lamb Chili*

15. *Beef Chili*

16. *Chicken Chili*

17.   Pegan Quinoa Salad and Baked Tuna

18.   Sweet Potato Gnocchi in an Herbed Dairy-Free Sauce

19.   Pegan Cauliflower Gnocchi in a Creamy Sauce

20.   Crispy Baked Chicken with Sweet Potato and Broccoli Tots

21.   Mexican Sweet Tater Tots with Coconut-Cinnamon Pork Chops

Chapter 7.   Protein Main Courses

22.   Miso-Glazed Pan-Seared Salmon with Bok Choy

23.   Smoked Salmon, Cucumber, and Avocado Sushi

24.   Oil-Poached Whitefish with Lemony Gremolata

25.   Ceviche Fish Tacos with Easy Guacamole

26.   Shrimp Scampi with Baby Spinach

27.   Shrimp Fried Rice

28.   Mussels with Lemon-Garlic-Herb Broth

29.   Clam Linguine with Zucchini Noodles

30.   Crab Cakes with Creamy Citrus Slaw

31.   Peppery Shrimp and Steak for Two

32.   Creamy Salmon Capers with Spiralled Zoodles

33.   Garlicky Fish Fillets with Parsley leaves

34.   Easy Butter Shrimp Scampi with Parsley Leaves

35.   One pan Broiled Salmon with Yellow Miso

36.   Garlic and Herb Mussels in Rose Broth

37.   Spicy Crabs with Chilled Coleslaw Mix

38.   Coconut Salmon with Scallion Greens

39.   Soy dipped Avocado Sushi Roll

40.   Baked Garlic marinade Arctic char Fillets

41.   Spicy Cilantro Fish wrapped in Lettuce Leaves

42.   Homemade Shrimp and Pea Bowl with Cashews

43. *Mussel Spinach Cold Butter Bowl*

44. *Creamy Zucchini Clam Shallow Bowls*

45. *Chicken Mushroom Shrimp Mix with Green Onions*

Chapter 8.   Appendix Measurement Conversions

Volume Equivalents (Liquid)

Volume Equivalents (Dry)

Oven Temperatures

Conclusion

Introduction

"The Pegan Diet" is a special low carb, high protein, and low-fat diet that allows you to lose weight quickly and easily and improve your health. This regimen is divided into two phases. In the first phase, it allows you to lose weight and eliminate your bad habits, and in the second phase, it helps you do the maintenance, which will enable you to maintain optimum nutrition. When following a Pegan diet, every meal will be delicious, and you will not have cravings anymore.

The diet helps you lose weight quickly because it does not require you to work out or change your eating habits. Just adjusting the quantity of food you eat will allow you to lose weight quickly and efficiently.

The Pegan diet has been proven to work for people looking to lose weight and improve their health.

Thanks to the Pegan diet, you will improve your health and appearance. Moreover, being calorically restricted means that you will have more energy throughout the day. In turn, this will make it uncomplicated for you to exercise regularly or work out at the gym!

Chapter 1.   What is the Pegan Diet?

The pegan diet is a dieting principle that adheres to the paleo and vegan diets, which is based on the idea that nutrient-dense, whole foods are capable of reducing inflammation, moderate blood sugar level, and as well provide optimal health.

Like many, you may have concluded that following the paleo and vegan, at the same time, will not be possible; this expert says it is pretty understandable.

You may have read or heard certain persons talk about their personal experiences while on the Pegan Diet. How fascinating was it? Instead, did you find such stories a little odd?

The pegan diet helps improve one's health in many ways. One of the most vital points of the pegan diet is the greater emphasis on eating actual vegetables and fruits, some of the most nutrient-dense and diverse foods people can eat. This incorporates a lot of fiber, vitamins, minerals, and plant compounds in one's diet. Also, the pegan diet focuses on increasing healthy fats from fish, nuts, seeds, and other plants, which positively impact one's health, especially heart health. Furthermore, the emphasis on whole foods and sustainably sourced foods reduces processed foods and improves overall diet quality.

Pegan Diet is a special diet with a peculiar set of guidelines and is less restrictive than a paleo diet and the vegan diet.

It emphasizes eating vegetables and fruit and moderately consuming a certain amount of meat, fish, seeds, and nuts, with some legumes being inclusive.

Primarily processed oils, sugars, and grains are not permitted, as a matter of principle, though an intake of a minimal amount of this may not be an issue.

The pegan diet is not made as a typical, short-term diet. Instead, it directs to be more sustainable so that you can follow it indefinitely.

As such, one would be expected to be highly confused about the pegan diet, given its contradictory nature. However, what the pegan diet seeks to do is to combine certain principles from both diets, which will be discussed later. However, the general idea of the pegan diet is that one is supposed to eat nutrient-dense whole foods, which can reduce inflammation, balance blood sugar, allowing one to be at optimal health. As one would see that the pegan diet combines both vegan and paleo diets, both limited diets, one might think that this means that only the overlap between the two is allowed, which would result in a very, very limited diet indeed. However, contrary to this idea, it is even less restrictive than either vegan or paleo by themselves, as it seeks to combine principles, not the restrictions per se.

Many emphases are placed on eating fruits and vegetables, like the vegan diet, but unlike the vegan diet, animal proteins such as meats and fish are allowed, and some nuts, seeds, and legumes. Some items banned by both are permitted, such as oils and some processed sugars, but note that these should be highly restricted. The pegan diet is not a crash diet but rather a sustainable diet meant to be easy to stick to, allowing one to stay on it indefinitely rather than losing the willpower to continue later on.

What does this tell you?

The pegan diet, though standing on the paleo and vegan diets principles, still has its particular rubric that is made in such a way as to encourage sustainability over a long period.

As a rule, those on pegan diets is hoping to consume fruits and vegetables up to 75%; and 25% of other foods primarily divided among eggs, meats; healthy fats, like nuts and seeds, including also certain legumes and gluten-free whole grains that you can take in limited quantities.

Responsible source of protein

While this diet principle encourages more plant-based foods, enough animal protein consumption is advised.

Note also that as 75% of diets consist of vegetables and fruits, you're likely to have a reduced meat consumption compared to that of the average paleo diet, although more compared to any vegan diet.

This diet will not allow you to eat conventionally manufactured meats or eggs; instead, the emphasis is placed on grass-fed, pasture-raised foundations of beef, poultry, and pork; whole eggs too.

Low mercury content fish like wild salmon and sardines, in particular, is promoted as a better source of protein.

Chapter 2.　Vegan Diet and Workout: Benefits and Disadvantages

At this moment, everybody needs a piece of sound weight reduction achievement, and that's only the tip of the iceberg, and more individuals are attempting the Veggie lover Diet, otherwise called the Plant-Based Eating regimen. Dissimilar to keto eat fewer carbs, which are both difficult to maintain and not heart-solid over the long haul, the Vegetarian Diet is an entire food plant-based method of eating that is sound, practical, and offers insusceptibility boosting food varieties to keep your energy up and your protections solid against becoming ill, as you shed pounds.

A few weight control plans are flying around the web that incorporates the Adele Diet, otherwise called the Sir food Diet. (We attempted it, and this is what occurred.) At that point, there is Irregular Fasting. (Which additionally works, as long as you eat solid during the "on eating hours."?)

More individuals are attempting to eat plant-based than at any other time, at present: 23% of purchasers are consolidating plant-based or veggie lover food sources into their eating regimen: Deals of plant-based meats are up 35%, while generally, deals of all vegetarian food sources are up 90% since the tallness of the Coronavirus emergency. It's just developing, as individuals need an eating routine that allows them to get in shape and be sound. A veggie lover or plant-based "clean-eating" diet guarantees both: Solid resistance, in addition to consistent weight reduction.

Solid Weight reduction, less fatty Kid Arrangement With Plant-Based Protein

The Vegetarian Diet and Plant-Based Eating routine is winning now since it's more grounded than different eating regimens. Furthermore, indeed, it's by and large what it seems like. You avoid irritation boosting creature items and fill your plate with plant-based entire food varieties that are low in oil, negligibly cooked, and brimming with fiber. Also, prepare to have your mind blown. It works.

Yet, the explanation that the Veggie lover Diet is getting on right presently is two-crease: One is that individuals are avoiding meat during the hour of Coronavirus. The other is that the Vegetarian Diet causes you to get in shape and fabricate your insusceptibility. It's likewise reasonable, sound, and familiar. There isn't anything more regular than eating an entire food plant-based eating regimen low in oils and fats.

The Veggie lover Diet is by and large what it seems like: You eat vast loads of vegetables, natural products, vegetables, grains, nuts, and seeds. There's no point framework or tallying carbs, calories, or net carbs. You fill your plate with plant-based whole food sources that are low in oil, negligibly cooked, and brimming with fiber. If you can develop it, it's a "Go!" On the off chance that you need to search for fixings on a mark and there are many, it's an "Off limits!" This primary method of getting in shape is standard, automatic, and feasible. On the off chance that you shed 2 pounds every week (which is a solid rate), you can shed 12 pounds by the fourth of July.

The Veggie Lover Diet for Weight Reduction Is Famous During Coronavirus

For what reason is the Veggie lover Diet having a second? Above all else, meat handling plants are as yet overflowing with Coronavirus and simply this week, Tyson had to close down its most extraordinary pork plant as one-fifth of the labor force, or 555 of the specialists) tried positive for the infection. This implies that store network interferences guarantee to drive up the expense of meats, and customers are apprehensive that meat could spread the condition, even though there is no proof that this has occurred at this point.

Then, on the potential gain, the Vegetarian Diet is typical, permitting the calorie counter to top off on vegetables and vegetables, grains and nuts and seed, in addition to the organic product - all food varieties that are brimming with fiber, satisfyingly filling and offer a lot of dietary protein. For the food varieties that provide the most protein, see this rundown. For most calorie counters, getting sufficient protein on a vegetarian diet begins with a bowl of oats and plant-based milk, which gets you around one-fourth of the path. There is a simple, low-calory feast.

Why the Veggie Lover Diet Works: Fiber Is a Weight Watcher's Distinct Advantage to Shed Fat

To top off on good food sources, the higher the fiber content, the better. Fiber has been given unfavorable criticism as a "controller" for any individual who experiences difficulty going to the restroom. However, it's the "counter carb" regarding eating quality food sources that prod weight reduction. When people with diabetes are put on a strict low-carb diet, they are instructed to search for fiber since the fiber-to-carb proportion is a higher priority than carbs alone. This is why an organic product, however higher in carbs than vegetables, doesn't make you fat.

The fiber in the food you eat permits the body to get to sound supplements while keeping glucose low and your insulin reaction under control. The lower your glucose, the lower your insulin reaction, and the less your body gets the sign to store the additional energy as fat.

The high-fiber substance of foods grown from the ground implies that the "net carb" impact offers every one of the supplements less of the calories, carbs, and unfortunate fat that creature items or profoundly prepared food sources convey. The way to get in shape on the Veggie lover Diet is to pick food sources that are as near nature develops them as expected. Entire food varieties that are plant-based, including vegetables, organic products, vegetables, nuts, seeds, and grains, make up a solid combination of nutrients and minerals, proteins, and complex carbs to cause the individual eating this approach to feel fulfilled and complete, never ravenous and denied, and still get in shape.

At the point when your fat admission is low - which means no creature fat and negligible oils - your body will prepare prepared energy based on what is put away in the body. You go through your glycogen first, and as anybody probably is aware who has required a 45-minute twist class or run, you switch over your energy framework when you run out of accessible put-away energy in the muscles and the liver, and afterward begin to consume off fat stores and haul point out of capacity. The Vegetarian Diet low in oils is a usual method to provoke your body to discover energy from the inside, basically firing up your motors to copy fat quicker.

Stay Sound as You Get thinner With Invulnerable Boosting Vegetables and Natural products.

The Veggie lover Diet is loaded with vegetables and organic products that offer resistance-boosting properties. Every one of the food sources known to help support your normal invulnerability is "on the rundown" for the Vegetarian Diet. Broccoli, mushrooms, peppers, and citrus belong to the 13 food varieties that offer the most resistance per chomp.

The Veggie lover Diet can help you get in shape that is reasonable by limiting eating prepared food varieties that will probably be high in added sugar and fat, low in fiber, and brimming with added substances. So while potato chips are, for the most part, vegetarian, they don't cut since they are prepared. The equivalent goes for Twizzlers and other bundled food sources that are just vegetarian since they don't contain creature items. To get fit, you need to think, "On the off chance that I can develop it, I can eat it." You have never seen a PopTart in a nursery.

When you eat the Veggie lover Diet, you get more fit since you avoid aggravation boosting creature items and fill your plate with plant-based entire food varieties that are low in oil, evidently cooked, and brimming with fiber. What's more, prepare to be blown away. It works. You can let go up to 2 to 3 pounds per week and keep it off if you adhere to an entire food plant-based – or vegetarian diet.

Chapter 3.   Paleo Diet and Workout: Benefits and Disadvantages

The Paleo diet is not about a pure diet designed to lose weight quickly in the shortest possible time. Instead, it is a form of nutrition that can be pursued over the long term. Of course, the Paleo Diet can help you lose weight. However, this is not the primary goal of this type of diet.

The Paleo Diet has many advantages and positive effects on the body:

Protection against civilization diseases:

The risk of civilization diseases is reduced. Instead, one learns again to listen to the body's needs and thus intuitively feed it the food it needs to function smoothly. Many people notice a positive effect on the body relatively quickly after changing their diet. You feel fitter, more powerful, and more balanced.

There is no risk of malnutrition:

As no nutrients are foregone with the Paleo diet, there is no risk that the body could lack certain nutrients. Our body needs all three macronutrients: carbohydrates, fats, and proteins. In contrast to other diets, all three macronutrients are allowed to be included. Thus, the body is not limited in its functionality but is supported.

No starvation as with other diets:

Many diets are based on strict calorie restrictions. This is not the case here. You don't have to count calories. Instead, your diet is based on healthy and wholesome foods. In contrast to finished products, for example, these automatically keep you full longer. Accordingly, you do not need to consume tons of calories. You will find yourself back to a healthy feeling of hunger and satiety.

No yo-yo effect: The notorious yo-yo effect does not occur with the Paleo diet either. The yo-yo effect is created by restricting the number of calories. If these are limited over a more extended period, the body and the metabolism fall into starvation mode. This means that the metabolism slows down and requires less energy overall. If the restriction is lifted again and more energy is supplied to the body in calories, then there is an excess of energy. Since the body cannot use the power, it stores it as fat cells in the body.

Consumption of wholesome and healthy foods:

A wholesome, healthy, and natural diet supplies the body with all the essential macronutrients and all the crucial vitamins and minerals. The body also needs these so that it can maintain all functions. Simultaneously, healthy and natural foods strengthen our immune system, and we are less susceptible to diseases. If you eat a balanced diet within the Paleo diet, you don't have to worry about a deficiency symptom. All critical vitamins and minerals are adequately covered.

Fit and high-performance:

Many are probably familiar with the well-known lunchtime low that always spreads after lunch and lays paralyzing over you. In general, constant tiredness is part of everyday life for many people. You feel unbalanced and unmotivated. Few, however, an associate diet with performance. As the motto goes: You are what you eat! When switching to Paleo, many users experience a real boost in performance. You are suddenly full of energy and motivation. The afternoon tiredness is also blown away. This is a clear sign that your body feeds on healthy foods and can use them optimally for you.

Interesting facts about the Paleo Diet:

Cooking healthily every day is, of course, relatively time-consuming. The fresh ingredients need to be processed and cooked. The planning of the dishes and the shopping will probably take longer than usual. Many have to get used to this change first. We live in a time when all should go quickly—cooking and eating too. But it is an investment in your own body and your health. To save time, I recommend that you pre-cook 2-3 times a week for several days. So you don't have to cook fresh every day, but you can freshen up the portions the next day. You can also freeze more significant portions wonderfully.

The Paleo diet is about taking foods that are of high quality. That means wild fish, organic meat, organic eggs, and organic fruit and vegetables. After all, it would be best if you eat as naturally as possible. Sustainability is also an important aspect. Sustainability, health, and factory farming do not go together. In the long run, this can have an impact on your wallet. Here I can recommend comparing different producers and suppliers to find out where you can get the best price-performance ratio. To do this, you should combine the various dishes in such a way that you only need a few different foods.

Chapter 4.   The Importance of Nutrients: Where Do Vegans and Paleos Get Proteins, Fat, Carbs, Sugar and Fibers

Pegan diet, or Pegan, could be an eating routine that comprises exceptionally low carbs and high fat. How a few weight control plans are there where you can start your downtime with bacon and eggs, heaps of it, and follow it up with chicken wings for lunch and steak and broccoli for supper. That may sound unrealistic for some. This eating regimen is regularly an incredible day of eating, and you followed the establishments consummately with that feast set up. When you take a low amount of carbs, your body gets place into a territory of Pegan. What this proposes is your body consumes fat for energy. Are you still confused about initiating this dietary program? You are not sure of what you can eat and what should be avoided or limited. Let us help you with these recommendations.

Anyway, it is a sure thing to remain under 25 net carbs. A few would propose that when no doubt about its acceptance is the point you are genuinely placing your body into Pegan, you should keep underneath ten net carbs. On the chance that you don't know what net carbs are, let me encourage you. Web carbs are the number of carbs you eat short of the amount of dietary fiber. Along these lines, if you eat a sum of 35 grams of web carbs and thirteen grams of dietary fiber, your net carbs for the day would be 22. Sufficiently simple, isn't that so?

All in all, other than weight reduction, what else is sweet about Pegan? Numerous people talk concerning their improved mental clearness when on the eating regimen. Another benefit has an ascent in energy. One more is a diminished craving. One factor to worry over when happening the Pegan diet is something many refer to as Pegan influenza. Not every person encounters this; aside from this that does it tends to be intense. You can feel torpid, and you may have a migraine. It won't keep going exceptionally long. When you think this way, verify you get masses of water and rest to initiate through it. On the off chance that this seems as though the sort of diet you would be interested in, at that point, what are you anticipating? Jump heard first into Pegan. You won't accept the outcomes you get in a concise amount of time.

Carbohydrates:

It would be best to give up polished rice in favor of brown rice, albeit limiting it to just half a cup per meal. Other sources of carbohydrates could include regular potatoes, parsnips, black rice (half-a-cup per meal), Winter Squash, Spaghetti Squash, Acorn Squash, plantains, sweet potatoes, coconut flour, almond flour, Quinoa (half-a-cup per meal), pumpkins, wild rice (half-a-cup per meal), coconut floor, Yam Noodles – Shirataki, etc. Always ensure that your glycemic load remains within normal levels. This means that a healthy sugar-insulin balance should be witnessed in your bloodstream. Otherwise, you place your heart, kidneys, liver, etc., at risk for life-threatening illnesses.

Fats:

It may amaze you to know that popular oils like soybean oil, canola oil, sunflower oil, and corn oil are detrimental to your health. Soybean oil contains Omega-6 fats, which are responsible for inflammation; this oil undergoes high processing. It would be better to go in for coconut oil, sesame seed oil, avocado oil, olive oil, and Macadamia nut oil. They contain Omega-3 fats, which are excellent for your heart and cholesterol levels. Yes, you may even find Omega-3 fatty acids in meat obtained from grass-fed livestock or sustainably raised animals. However, your consumption of these saturated fats should remain low. Other products containing healthy fats are salmon, sardines, coconut milk, avocado, goat cheese, cashew butter, grass-fed butter, and almond butter. As for seeds and nuts, you may add flax seeds, sesame seeds, hemp seeds, chia seeds, pumpkin seeds, walnuts, almonds, pistachios, and cashews to your diet.

Sugar:

It would be greater to regard it as an occasional treat from the time you begin your Pegan diet. For instance, stop sprinkling large amounts of sugar on every recipe, over-sweetening your coffee and tea, eating sugary condiments, and gorging on sugary cereals. It is not essential what form the sugar is in; it is still not healthy. Instead, go in for coconut sugar, organic honey, or raw maple syrup as substitutes, albeit in reasonable amounts. Since they are not incredibly processed, they are safer for your health.

Chapter 5.   What can a Pegan eat and What Cannot?

Are you sure you're ready to start the pegan diet? Perhaps you have alerted your relatives (household members) about your newfound diet to prepare them for this carb-reduction diet? Let me not bother you with the headache, irritability, uncontrollable fatigue, and cravings often associated with removing carbs from one's diet. You could try creating a couple of days' worth of a meal plan, with a grocery inventory patterned to take care of the recipes you will need.

Healthiest diet

Those who want to know why the pegan diet is becoming popular in recent times will interest you to know that it's among the healthiest diets scientifically proven to be effective.

Just recently, a study came out suggesting the first five healthiest foods to include: the Low-carb, whole-food diet that is promoted chiefly for people who want to lose weight and reduce the risk of disease infection for optimum health; the Mediterranean diet, the Paleo diet, the Vegan diet, and the Gluten-free diet.

Foods to eat while on the Pegan Diet

As you would soon find out, the pegan diet strongly promotes those whole foods or those foods that do not undergo much or no processing at all before you eat them. As you have guessed already, that is why plants seem to have a more significant stake in the pegan diet.

As a matter of principle, you're advised to eat lots of plants as a primary food source: thus vegetables and fruits, amounting to 75% of your total food consumption within the period.

Low-glycemic fruits and vegetables, like non-starchy vegetables, berries, and the likes, are encouraged to reduce once blood sugar reaction.

A small quantity of starchy vegetables and sweet fruits is often permitted for people that have achieved a healthy blood sugar regulation before commencing the diet.

As stated earlier, the healthy protein source should be a significant part of the remaining 25 % of your food consumption after removing 75% for fruits and vegetables.

Again, you're expected to maintain minimally processed fats, otherwise refers to as healthy fats from foods sources like:

- The Nuts- excluding peanuts
- The Seeds- excluding refined seed oils
- The Avocados and the olives- including cold-pressed olive and avocado oils
- The Coconut- unrefined coconut oil is also allowed
- The Omega-3s- with emphasis on the low-mercury fish or algae

You may also consider pasture-raised meats and whole eggs for the fat content of your pegan diet.

You can take selected whole grains and legumes, especially the gluten-free whole grains and legumes but in a minimal amount; most of this kind of food is prohibited because of their role in influencing blood sugar.

Grain intake is estimated not to exceed a 1/2 cup or 125 grams in every meal, just as legume is kept below 1 cup or 75 grams each meal, respectively.

Few grains and legumes that you may consider eating will include:

Black rice, millet, quinoa, teff, oats, and amaranth- for grains

Black beans, lentils, pinto beans, and chickpeas- for legumes

Diabetes patients or related medical condition patients that encourage poor blood sugar regulation should keep away from grains and legumes.

Bottom of Form

Pegan Diet, Food to Avoid

Those who want to go with the pegan diet should understand its principles and know those foods that are not allowed or at most are discouraged because of their nutritional content or relative response it evokes in the body.

Things like:

- Sugar
- Gluten
- Dairy
- Canola, soybean, corn oils, or grape seed

Anything that has encountered certain chemical additives like pesticides, hormones, dyes, GMOs, artificial sweeteners, antibiotics, and preservatives, should not be consumed.

As a general Rule on this Diet, you're advised to at all times do the following:

Reduce starchy veggies in your meal, e.g., potatoes or the winter squash, to something less than 1/2 cup in a day while also consuming only the lower-sugar fruits like the berries and kiwi. If you must eat beans, it should be limited to something less than a cup daily.

Whole grains that do not have gluttons like teff, black rice, quinoa, and amaranth should also be eaten cautiously, with something less than 1/2 cup in each meal.

Once in a while, you may take honey or sugar in the form of maple syrup.

You may also eat once in a while grass-fed, organic dairy products like ghee or kefir. When there are no adverse result reports in terms of discomfort, milk product of sheep and goats may also be taken.

Every food taken should be modestly processed with a significant part of its natural content still intact.

Although the pegan diet does not explicitly mention alcohol, the paleo diet forbids it..

Chapter 6.   Protein Dinner

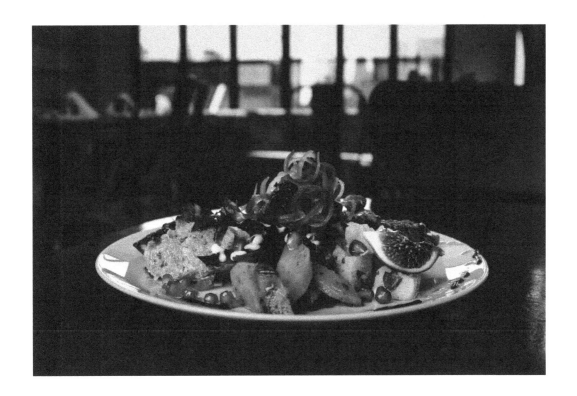

1. Belgian Endive Frittata

Preparation Time: 10 Minutes

Cooking Time: 20 Minutes

Servings: 2

Ingredients:

- 1/2 lb. Belgian endive
- 1 tablespoon olive oil
- 1/2 red onion
- 1/4 tsp. salt
- 2 oz. cheddar cheese
- 1 garlic clove
- 1/4 tsp. dill

Directions:

1. In a bowl whisk eggs with salt and cheese
2. In a frying pan heat olive oil and pour egg mixture
3. Add remaining ingredients and mix well
4. Serve when ready

Nutrition:

Calories: 354   Carbs: 34.6g

Fat: 20.7g   Fiber: 7g

Protein: 11g

2. Carrot Frittata

Preparation Time: 10 Minutes

Cooking Time: 20 Minutes

Servings: 2

Ingredients:

- 1/2 lb. carrot
- 1 tablespoon olive oil
- 1/2 red onion
- 1/4 tsp. salt
- 2 oz. cheddar cheese
- 1 garlic clove
- 1/4 tsp. dill

Directions:

1. In a bowl whisk eggs with salt and cheese
2. In a frying pan heat olive oil and pour egg mixture
3. Add remaining ingredients and mix well
4. Serve when ready

Nutrition:

Calories 83   Carbs: 3g

Fat: 5g   Fiber: 1g

Protein: 7g   Sodium: 385mg

3. Kale Frittata

Preparation Time: 10 Minutes

Cooking Time: 20 Minutes

Servings: 2

Ingredients:

- 1 cup kale
- 1 tablespoon olive oil
- 1/2 red onion
- 1/4 tsp. salt
- 2 oz. cheddar cheese
- 1 garlic clove
- 1/4 tsp. dill

Directions:

1. In a skillet sauté kale until tender
2. In a bowl whisk eggs with salt and cheese
3. In a frying pan heat olive oil and pour egg mixture
4. Add remaining ingredients and mix well
5. When ready serve with sautéed kale

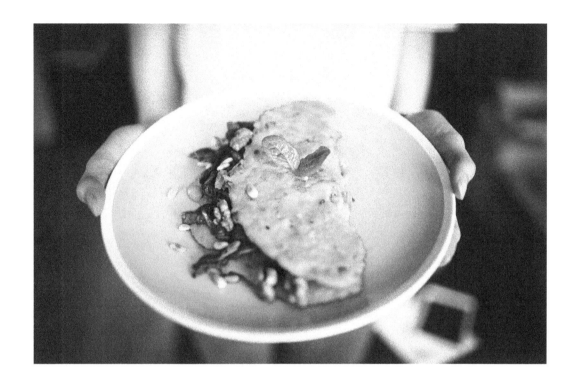

Nutrition:

Calories 83   Carbs: 3g

Fat: 5g   Fiber: 1g

Protein: 7g   Sodium: 385mg

4. Ham Frittata

Preparation Time: 10 Minutes

Cooking Time: 20 Minutes

Servings: 2

Ingredients:

- 8-10 slices ham
- 1 tablespoon olive oil
- 1/2 red onion
- 1/4 tsp. salt
- 2 oz. parmesan cheese
- 1 garlic clove
- 1/4 tsp. dill

Directions:

1. In a bowl whisk eggs with salt and parmesan cheese
2. In a frying pan heat olive oil and pour egg mixture
3. Add remaining ingredients and mix well
4. When the ham and eggs are cooked remove from heat and serve

Nutrition:

Calories: 83   Carbs: 3g

Fat: 5g   Fiber: 1g

Protein: 7g   Sodium: 385mg

5. Broccoli Frittata

Preparation Time: 10 Minutes

Cooking Time: 20 Minutes

Servings: 2

Ingredients:

- 1 cup broccoli
- 1 tablespoon olive oil
- 1/2 red onion
- 1/4 tsp. salt
- 2 oz. cheddar cheese
- 1 garlic clove
- 1/2 tsp. dill

Directions:

1. In a skillet sauté broccoli until tender
2. In a bowl whisk eggs with salt and cheese
3. In a frying pan heat olive oil and pour egg mixture
4. Add remaining ingredients and mix well
5. When ready serve with sautéed broccoli

Nutrition:

Calories: 83

Carbs: 3g

Fat: 5g

Fiber: 1g

Protein: 7g

Sodium: 385mg

6. Apple Slaw

Preparation Time: 5 Minutes

Cooking Time: 0 Minutes

Servings: 2

Ingredients:

- 4 cups cabbage
- 2 cups apples
- 1/4 cup Greek Yogurt
- 2 tablespoons honey
- 1/4 tsp. salt

Directions:

1. In a bowl mix all ingredients and mix well
2. Serve with dressing

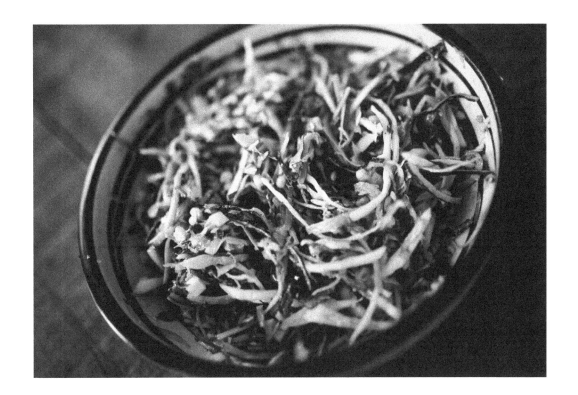

Nutrition:

Calories 60

Carbs: 3g

Fat: 5g

Fiber: 30g

7. Ground Beef with Peas

Preparation Time: 15 Minutes

Cooking Time: 40 Minutes

Servings: 6

Ingredients:

- 2 tablespoons olive oil
- 1 pound grass-fed lean ground beef
- 1 large onion, chopped finely
- 2 garlic cloves, minced
- 1/2 tablespoon fresh ginger, minced
- 1 teaspoon ground coriander
- 1 teaspoon ground cumin
- 1/4 teaspoon chili powder
- 2 medium tomatoes, seeded and chopped
- 1/2 cup homemade chicken broth
- Salt and ground black pepper, as required
- 21/4 cups fresh peas, shelled
- 2 tablespoons fresh cilantro, chopped

Directions:

1. In a large skillet, heat the oil over medium heat and cook the beef for about 4-5 minutes or until browned completely.
2. With a slotted spoon, transfer the beef into a large bowl.
3. In the same skillet, add onion and sauté for about 4-6 minutes.
4. Add the garlic, ginger, coriander, cumin and chili powder and sauté for about 1 minute.
5. Add the tomatoes and cook for about 2-3 minutes, crushing completely with the back of spoon.
6. Stir in the beef and broth and bring to a boil.

7. Reduce the heat to medium-low and simmer, covered for about 8-10 minutes, stirring occasionally.
8. Stir in peas and cook for 10-15 minutes.
9. Remove from heat and serve hot with the garnishing of almonds and cilantro leaves.

Nutrition:

Calories: 243   Carbs: 12.7g

Tot Fat: 11.9g   Saturated Fat: 3.8g

Protein: 19.5g

8. Beef with Lentils

Preparation Time: 15 Minutes

Cooking Time: 50 Minutes

Servings: 6

Ingredients:

- 3 tablespoons extra-virgin olive oil, divided
- 1 onion, chopped
- 1 tablespoon fresh ginger, minced
- 4 garlic cloves, minced
- 3 plum tomatoes, chopped finely
- 2 cups dried red lentils, soaked for 30 minutes and drained
- 2 cups homemade chicken broth
- 2 teaspoons cumin seeds
- 1/2 teaspoon cayenne pepper
- 1 pound grass-fed lean ground beef
- 1 jalapeño pepper, seeded and chopped
- 2 scallions, chopped

Directions:

1. In a Dutch oven, heat 1 tablespoon of oil over medium heat and sauté the onion, ginger and garlic for about 5 minutes.
2. Stir in the tomatoes, lentils and broth and bring to a boil
3. Reduce the heat to medium-low and simmer, covered for about 30 minutes.
4. Meanwhile, in a skillet, heat remaining oil over medium heat.
5. Add the cumin seeds and sauté for about 30 seconds.
6. Add the paprika and sauté for about 30 seconds.
7. Transfer the mixture into a small bowl and set aside.
8. In the same skillet, add the beef and cook for about 4-5 minutes.
9. Add jalapeño and scallion and cook for about 4-5 minutes.

10. Add the spiced oil mixture and stir to combine well.
11. Transfer the beef mixture into the simmering lentils and simmer for about 10-15 minutes or until desired doneness.
12. Serve hot.

Nutrition:

Calories: 469

Carbs: 45.1g

Tot Fat: 13,3g

Saturated Fat: 3.1g

Fiber: 21.1g

Protein: 42.3g

9. Beef with Cauliflower

Preparation Time: 15 Minutes

Cooking Time: 12 Minutes

Servings: 4

Ingredients:

- 1 tablespoon coconut oil
- 4 garlic cloves, minced
- 1 pound grass-fed beef sirloin steak, cut into bite-sized pieces
- 3 1/2 cups cauliflower florets
- 3 tablespoons coconut aminos
- 1/4 cup fresh cilantro leaves, chopped

Directions:

1. In a large skillet, heat the oil over medium heat and sauté the garlic for about 1 minute.
2. Add beef and stir to combine.
3. Increase the heat to medium-high and cook for about 6-8 minutes or until browned from all sides.
4. Meanwhile, in a pan of boiling filtered water, add cauliflower and cook for about 5-6 minutes.
5. Drain the cauliflower completely.
6. Add the cauliflower and coconut aminos in skillet with beef and cook for about 2-3 minutes.
7. Serve with the garnishing of cilantro.

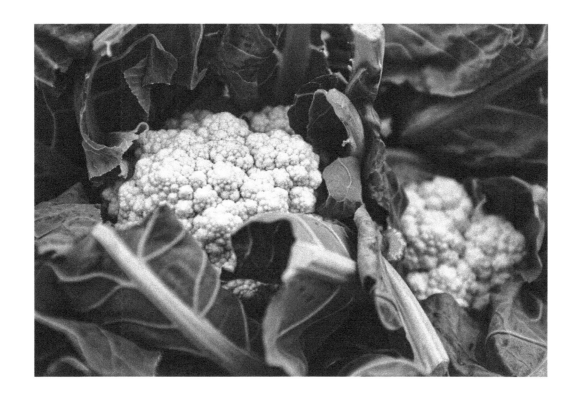

Nutrition:

Calories: 278   Carbs: 7.9g

Tot Fat: 10.6g   Saturated Fat: 5.6g

Sugar: 2.1g   Fiber: 2.3g

Protein: 36.3g

10. Glazed Flank Steak

Preparation Time: 15 Minutes

Cooking Time: 12 Minutes

Servings: 4

Ingredients:

- 2 tablespoons arrowroot flour
- Salt and ground black pepper, as required
- 1 pound grass-fed flank steak, cut into 1/4-inch thick slices
- 1/2 cup plus 1 tablespoon coconut oil, divided
- 2 garlic cloves, minced
- 1 teaspoon ground ginger
- Pinch of red pepper flakes, crushed
- 1/3 cup raw honey
- 1/2 cup homemade beef broth
- 1/2 cup coconut aminos
- 3 scallions, chopped

Directions:

1. In a bowl, add the arrowroot flour, salt and black pepper and mix well.
2. Coat the beef slices with arrowroot flour mixture evenly.
3. Shake off the excess arrowroot flour mixture and set aside for about 10-15 minutes.
4. For sauce: in a pan, melt 1 tablespoon of coconut oil over medium heat and sauté the garlic, ginger powder and red pepper flakes for about 1 minute.
5. Add the honey, broth and coconut aminos and stir to combine well.
6. Now, increase the heat to high and cook for about 3 minutes, stirring continuously.
7. Remove from the heat and set aside.
8. In a large skillet, melt the remaining coconut oil over medium heat and stir fry the beef for about 2-3 minutes.

9. Remove the oil from skillet and stir fry for about 1 minute.

10. Stir in the honey sauce and cook for about 3 minutes.

11. Stir in the scallion and cook for about 1 minute more.

12. Serve hot.

Nutrition:

Calories: 586

Carbs: 31.6g

Tot Fat: 36.9g

Saturated Fat: 27.5g

Fiber: 0.5g

Protein: 32.8g

Sugar: 23.6g

11. Stuffed Turkey Breast

Preparation Time: 20 Minutes

Cooking Time: 2 Hours

Servings: 12

Ingredients:

For Turkey Rub

- 1 (5-pound) whole, bone-in turkey breast
- 2 tablespoons fresh thyme leaves, chopped
- 2 tablespoons fresh rosemary, chopped
- 2 tablespoons olive oil

For Stuffing

- 1 small onion, thinly sliced
- 1 apple, peeled and thinly sliced
- 1 pear, peeled and thinly sliced
- 1/4 cup dried cranberries

For Glaze

- 2 cups fresh apple juice, divided
- 1 tablespoon olive oil
- 1 tablespoon brown mustard
- 1/2 tablespoon coconut sugar

Directions:

1. Preheat the oven to 325 degrees F. Arrange a rack in a roasting pan.
2. Arrange turkey breast into the prepared roasting pan, skin-side up.
3. With your fingers, gently loosen the skin from the meat, making deep pockets between the skin and meat.
4. For rub: in a small bowl, mix together fresh herbs and oil.

5. Rub half of herb mixture on the meat and then, spread the remaining paste evenly over the top of the skin.
6. For stuffing: in a bowl, mix together all ingredients.
7. Stuff each pocket with the stuffing mixture.
8. In the bottom of roasting pan, pour 1 cup of apple juice.
9. Roast for about 13/4-2 hours. (If skin becomes brown during roasting, then cover the pan with a piece of foil).
10. Meanwhile, for glaze: in a pan, add remaining apple juice, oil, mustard and brown sugar and bring to a boil.
11. Reduce the heat and simmer until thick glaze is formed.
12. In the last 30 minutes of cooking, coat turkey breast with glaze evenly.
13. Remove from oven and cut turkey into desired slices before serving.

Nutrition:

Calories: 290

Carbs: 19.1g

Tot Fat: 9.2g

Saturated Fat: 1.5g

Fiber: 2.4g

Protein: 32.5g

Sugar: 14.5g

12. Grilled Chicken Breast

Preparation Time: 15 Minutes

Cooking Time: 20 Minutes

Servings: 4

Ingredients:

- 1 (1-inch) piece fresh ginger, minced
- 2 garlic cloves, minced
- 1 cup fresh pineapple juice
- 1/4 cup coconut aminos
- 1/4 cup extra-virgin olive oil
- 1 teaspoon ground cinnamon
- 1 teaspoon ground cumin
- Salt, as required
- 4 grass-fed skinless, boneless chicken breasts

Directions:

1. In a large Ziploc bag add all ingredients and seal it.
2. Shake the bag to coat the chicken with marinade well.
3. Refrigerate to marinade for about 1 hour.
4. Preheat the grill to medium-high heat. Grease the grill grate.
5. Place the chicken breasts onto the grill and cook for about 10 minutes per side.
6. Serve hot.

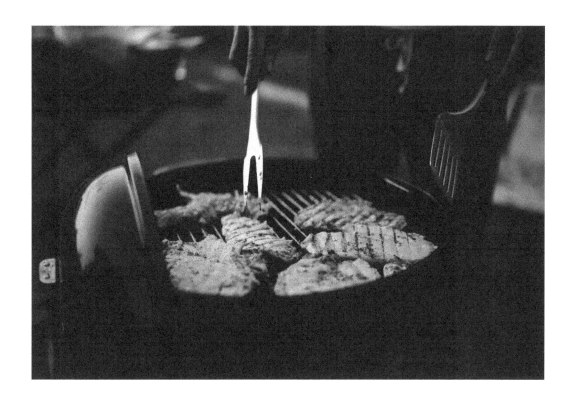

Nutrition:

Calories: 341

Carbs: 12.6g

Tot Fat: 17.9g

Saturated Fat: 3.7g

Fiber: 0.6g

Protein: 32.1g

Sugar: 6.3g

13. Glazed Chicken Thighs

Preparation Time: 10 Minutes

Cooking Time: 20 Minutes

Servings: 6

Ingredients:

- 3 garlic cloves, minced
- 1/2 cup fresh orange juice
- 1 tablespoon apple cider vinegar
- 2 tablespoons coconut aminos
- 1/2 teaspoon orange blossom water
- 1/4 teaspoon ground ginger
- 1/4 teaspoon ground cinnamon
- Salt, as required
- 2 pounds grass-fed skinless, bone-in chicken thighs

Directions:

1. For marinade: in a large bowl, place all ingredients except chicken and mix well.
2. Add the chicken and coat with marinade generously.
3. Cover the bowl of chicken and refrigerate for about 2 hours.
4. Remove the chicken from bowl, reserving marinade.
5. Heat a large nonstick wok, over medium-high heat and cook the chicken for about 5-6 minutes or until golden brown.
6. Flip the side and cook for about 4 minutes.
7. Add the reserved marinade and bring to a boil.

8. Now, reduce the heat to medium-low heat and cook, covered for about 6-8 minutes or until sauce becomes thick.
9. Serve hot.

Nutrition:

Calories: 305

Carbs: 8.3g

Tot Fat: 11.3g

Saturated Fat: 3.1g

Fiber: 0.1g

Protein: 44g

Sugar: 1.8g

14. Lamb Chili

Preparation Time: 15 Minutes

Cooking Time: 2 Hours

Servings: 6

Ingredients:

- 11/2 tablespoons extra-virgin olive oil, divided
- 1 cup onion, chopped
- 6 large garlic cloves, minced
- 2 dried New Mexico chills, stemmed, seeded and torn
- 3 dried ancho chills, stemmed, seeded and torn
- 2 teaspoons dried oregano, crushed
- 11/2 teaspoons ground cumin
- 2 large plum tomatoes, chopped
- 2 cups homemade chicken broth
- 1 pound grass-fed lamb stew meat, trimmed and cubed
- Salt and ground black pepper, as required
- 15 ounces cooked kidney beans

Directions:

1. In an oven-proof pan, heat 1 tablespoon of oil over medium heat and sauté the onion for about 4-5 minutes.
2. Add the garlic, both chills and spices and sauté for about 1 minute.
3. Add the tomatoes and broth and bring to a boil.
4. Reduce the heat to medium-low and simmer, covered for about 30 minutes.
5. Preheat the oven to 325 degrees F. Arrange a rack in the center of the oven.
6. Remove the pan from heat and set aside to cool slightly.
7. Transfer the chili mixture into a blender and pulse until pureed.
8. Return the puree in the same pan.

9. Meanwhile, in another pan, heat the remaining oil over medium-high heat and cook the lamb with salt and black pepper k for about 3-4 minutes.
10. Transfer the cooked lamb in the pan with puree and stir to combine.
11. Cover the pan and bake for about 50 minutes.
12. Remove pan from the oven and place over medium-low heat.
13. Simmer, uncovered for about 25 minutes.
14. Stir in kidney beans and simmer for about 5 minutes.
15. Serve hot.

Nutrition:

Calories: 430

Carbs: 49.7g

Tot Fat: 8.3g

Saturated Fat: 2.4g

Fiber: 12.4g

Protein: 40g

Sugar: 4.4g

15. Beef Chili

Preparation Time: 15 Minutes

Cooking Time: 2 Hours 15 Minutes

Servings: 8

Ingredients:

- 2 tablespoons extra-virgin olive oil
- 1 large onion, chopped
- 1 large green bell pepper, seeded and chopped
- 4 garlic cloves, minced
- 1 jalapeño pepper, chopped
- 1 teaspoon dried thyme, crushed
- 1 teaspoon dried basil, crushed
- 2 tablespoons red chili powder
- 1 tablespoon ground cumin
- 1 teaspoon ground allspice
- 2 pounds grass-fed lean ground beef
- 3 cups fresh tomatoes, chopped finely
- 2 cups homemade chicken broth
- 1 cup water

Directions:

1. In a large pan, heat the oil over medium heat and sauté the onion and bell pepper for about 5-7 minutes.
2. Add garlic, jalapeño pepper, herbs, spices and black pepper and sauté for about 1 minute.
3. Add the beef and cook for about 4-5 minutes.
4. Stir in the tomatoes and cook for about 2 minutes.
5. Add the broth and water and bring to a boil.
6. Reduce the heat to low and simmer, covered for about 2 hours.
7. Serve hot.

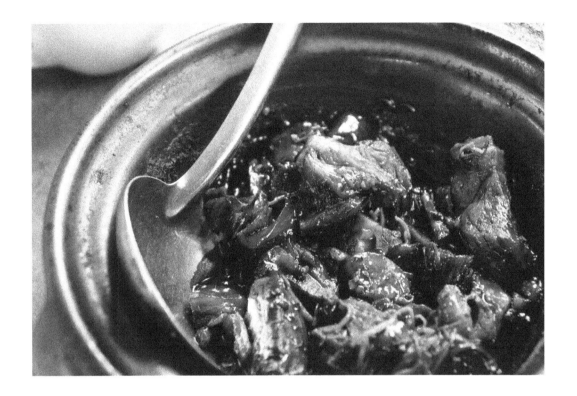

Nutrition:

Calories: 277

Carbs: 8g

Tot Fat: 14.6g

Saturated Fat: 5.2g

Protein: 25.7g

16. Chicken Chili

Preparation Time: 15 Minutes

Cooking Time: 40 Minutes

Servings: 6

Ingredients:

- 4 cups homemade chicken broth, divided
- 3 cups cooked black beans, divided
- 1 tablespoon extra-virgin olive oil
- 1 large onion, chopped
- 2 medium poblano peppers, seeded and chopped
- 1 jalapeño pepper, seeded and chopped
- 4 garlic cloves, minced
- 1 teaspoon dried thyme, crushed
- 11/2 tablespoons ground coriander
- 1 tablespoon ground cumin
- 1/2 tablespoon Ancho chili powder
- 4 cups grass-fed cooked chicken, shredded
- 1 tablespoon fresh lime juice
- 1/4 cup fresh cilantro, chopped

Directions:

1. In a food processor, add 1 cup of broth and 11/2 cups of black beans and pulse until smooth.
2. Transfer the beans puree into a bowl and set aside.
3. In a large pan, heat the oil over medium heat and sauté the onion, poblano and jalapeño for about 4-5 minutes.
4. Add the garlic, spices and sea salt and sauté for about 1 minute.
5. Add the beans puree and remaining broth and bring to a boil.

6. Reduce the heat to low and simmer for about 20 minutes.
7. Stir in the remaining beans, chicken and lime juice and bring to a boil.
8. Reduce the heat to low and simmer for about 5-10 minutes.
9. Serve hot with the topping of cilantro.

Nutrition:

Calories: 321

Carbs: 23.7g

Tot Fat: 7.4g

Saturated Fat: 1.4g

Fiber: 7g

Protein: 38.3g

Sugar: 2.4g

17. Pegan Quinoa Salad and Baked Tuna

Preparation Time: 10 Minutes

Cooking Time: 10 Minutes

Servings: 2

Ingredients:

- 2/3 cup quinoa, prepared ad directed
- 1/2 tablespoon red pepper infused olive oil
- 1/2 can organic whole kernel corn drained
- 3 pickled beets, quartered
- 1 teaspoon toasted coriander seeds
- 6 pickled jalapenos
- 1 ripe avocado peeled and sliced
- Juice of 1/2 lemon
- 2 filets tuna
- Salt and pepper
- 1/4 cup coconut oil

Directions:

1. Preheat broiler to hi and prepare 9x11 dish.
2. In Dutch oven combine olive oil, corn, pickled beets, toasted coriander seeds, pickled jalapenos. Toss with prepared quinoa and warm through.
3. Sprinkle Tunas with salt and pepper then brush both sides with coconut oil. Place under broiler 4-5 minute's per-side.

Nutrition:

Calories: 787   Tot Fat: 51.3g

Saturated Fat: 28.5g   Sodium: 284mg

Cholesterol: 38mg

18. Sweet Potato Gnocchi in an Herbed Dairy-Free Sauce

Preparation Time: 10 Minutes

Cooking Time: 15 Minutes

Servings: 2

Ingredients:

- 1 cup sweet potato mash
- 1/2 cup cassava or almond flour
- Olive oil
- 1 sprig parsley diced

Sauce

- 3 tablespoons unsalted butter or ghee
- 1 onion julienned
- 1 teaspoon garlic, minced
- 3/4 can coconut milk
- 2 teaspoons tapioca flour
- 2 teaspoons rosemary, diced
- 2 teaspoons Italian oregano, diced
- 1/3 teaspoon red pepper flakes
- 1 cup spinach or kale

Directions:

1. Mix sweet potato mash and flour together until smooth. Roll into 1-inch thick tube and cut into 4 pieces. Stick three in the refrigerator.
2. Cut each segment into 1-inch pieces and stick on baking tray. Drizzle with olive oil and pieces of parsley.
3. Boil pieces until they rise to the top.
4. Transfer gnocchi pieces to skillet and cook over medium heat 1 minute or until each side is a golden brown.

5. In skillet let butter melt them add julienned onions. Turn heat to medium-low and let onions sweat 10 minutes.

6. Whisk in garlic and coconut milk, stirring constantly for 30 seconds. Whisk in tapioca flour, diced rosemary, diced oregano, red pepper flakes. Bring to a low boil for 1-2 minutes constantly stirring.

7. Remove from heat and stir in spinach/kale

Nutrition:

Calories: 511   Tot Fat: 35g

Saturated Fat: 23.9g   Sodium: 71mg

Cholesterol: 15mg

19. Pegan Cauliflower Gnocchi in a Creamy Sauce

Preparation Time: 10 Minutes

Cooking Time: 55 Minutes

Servings: 4

Ingredients:

- 5 cups cauliflower, minced
- 1 cup cassava flour
- 1/2 teaspoon smoked paprika

Sauce

- 1 can coconut milk
- 5 cups spinach or kale
- 1 teaspoon garlic, minced
- 1/2 teaspoon lemon peel
- 1/3 teaspoon pepper
- 2 1/2 tablespoons tapioca flour

Directions:

1. Steam cauliflower 5-7 minutes, ring out water, put in blender along with cassava flour and smoked paprika. Blend until mix is smooth.
2. Roll dough into 1-inch thick tube then cut into four segments, place three in the refrigerator.
3. Cut each segment into 1-inch pieces, drop them into boiling water and let rise to surface.
4. Once they have risen, transfer them to baking tray 20 minutes, turn over, cook another 30 minutes.
5. In skillet over medium-high heat whisk together coconut milk, spinach or kale, minced garlic, lemon peel, pepper, tapioca flour. Stirring continuously until smooth and thickens.
6. Remove from heat and add in spinach or kale and gnocchi.

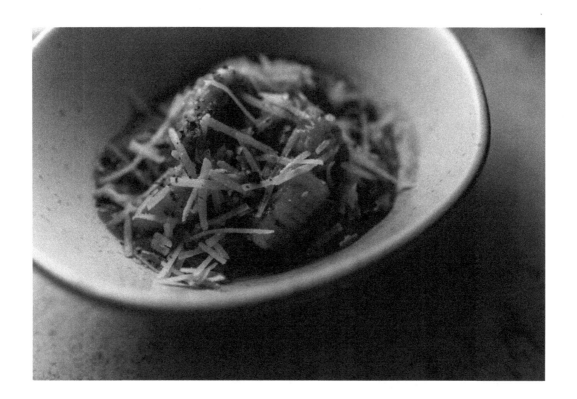

Nutrition:

Calories: 641

Tot Fat: 29.3g

Saturated Fat: 25.4g

Cholesterol: 0mg

Sodium 196mg

20. Crispy Baked Chicken with Sweet Potato and Broccoli Tots

Preparation Time: 10 Minutes

Cooking Time: 45 Minutes

Servings: 2

Ingredients:

- 2 3 oz. chicken patties
- 1 cup organic breadcrumbs or crushed cornflakes
- 2 cups sweet potato mash
- 2 cups broccoli mash
- 1 tablespoon paprika
- 1/2 tablespoon garlic powder and parsley

Directions:

1. Preheat oven to 425 and prepare medium sized baking dish.
2. Coat chicken patties with breadcrumbs, spray with olive oil, and bake 35-40 minutes.
3. Blend together sweet potato, broccoli, paprika, garlic powder and parsley.
4. Using hands form into tater tots and fry in coconut oil 2-3 minutes per side.

Nutrition:

Calories: 727   Tot Fat: 24g

Saturated Fat: 4.7g   Cholesterol: 45mg

Sodium: 1016mg

21. Mexican Sweet Tater Tots with Coconut-Cinnamon Pork Chops

Preparation Time: 10 Minutes

Cooking Time: 10 Minutes

Servings: 2

Ingredients:

- 1 tablespoon coconut oil
- 2 thin pork chops
- Cinnamon for sprinkling
- 4 cup sweet potato mash
- 1 tablespoon chili powder
- 1 tablespoon paprika
- 1 tablespoon cayenne pepper
- 1/2 tablespoon cumin
- 1/2 tablespoon garlic powder and parsley
- Coconut oil for frying OR olive oil infused with red pepper

Directions:

1. In skillet cook pork chops in coconut oil transfer to paper towel lined plates.
2. Mix together sweet potato, chili powder, paprika, cayenne powder, cumin, garlic powder & parsley.
3. With hands form into tater tots and fry in oil 2-3 minutes per side.
4. Before plating dust both sides of pork chops with cinnamon.

Nutrition:

Calories: 230   Tot Fat: 11.7g

Saturated Fat: 7.2g   Cholesterol: 60mg

Sodium: 275mg

Chapter 7.   Protein Main Courses

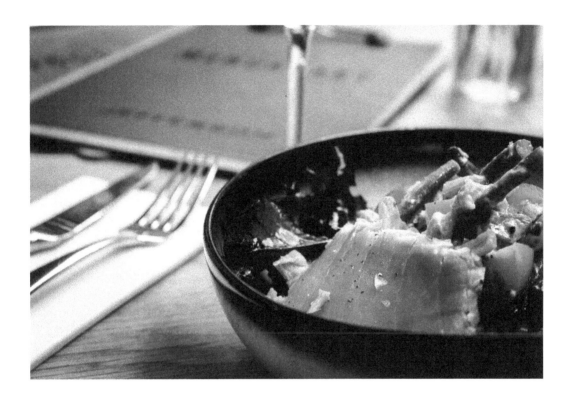

22. Miso-Glazed Pan-Seared Salmon with Bok Choy

Preparation time: 10 minutes

Cooking time: 15 minutes

Servings: 2

Ingredients:

- 2 (6-ounce) salmon fillets
- 1/4 cup white or yellow miso
- 2 tablespoons rice or coconut vinegar
- 2 tablespoons sesame oil, divided
- 1 tablespoon gluten-free soy sauce, tamari, or coconut aminos
- 1 tablespoon minced fresh ginger
- 1 clove garlic, minced
- 11/2 pounds (medium bunch) baby bok choy, core removed, sliced into 11/2-inch pieces, white stem and leafy green parts separated
- 2 tablespoons thinly sliced scallion whites (optional)
- 2 tablespoons thinly sliced scallion greens, for garnish (optional)

Directions:

1. Heat the broiler to high.
2. On a baking sheet or broiler pan, place the salmon, skin-side down, and pat it dry. In a small bowl, whisk together the miso, vinegar, 1 tablespoon of the sesame oil, the soy sauce, ginger, and garlic. Spread 2 tablespoons of the glaze evenly over the top of the salmon, setting aside the remainder. Let it stand for 10 minutes, if you have time.
3. Broil the salmon until the glaze is bubbly, 3 to 4 minutes. Cover it loosely with foil and continue to broil until slightly pink in the center, another 3 to 4 minutes. Remove the salmon from the broiler, remove the foil, and let it cool.

4. In a large skillet over medium-high heat, heat the remaining 1 tablespoon sesame oil. Add the bok choy stems and scallion whites (if using) and cook until just tender, 2 to 3 minutes. Stir in the remaining miso glaze and cook until fragrant, 30 to 60 seconds. Add the bok choy greens, cover, and steam until just wilted, 30 seconds. Toss to coat with the sauce.
5. To serve, divide the bok choy evenly between two plates. Top each with a salmon fillet and sprinkle with scallion greens (if using).

Nutrition:

Calories: 210

Carbs: 35.1g

Fat: 3.2g

Fiber: 13.7g

Protein: 12.2g

23. Smoked Salmon, Cucumber, and Avocado Sushi

Preparation time: 10 minutes

Cooking time: 15 minutes

Servings: 2

Ingredients:

- 2 sheets sushi nori
- 1 medium avocado, pitted and peeled
- 2 tablespoons sesame seeds, divided (optional)
- 4 ounces smoked salmon (about 4 thin slices)
- 1 medium cucumber, cut into matchsticks
- 3 tablespoons pickled ginger (optional)
- 1 teaspoon wasabi paste (optional)
- Gluten-free soy sauce, tamari, or coconut aminos, for dipping

Directions:

1. Lay 1 piece of nori on a sheet of parchment paper or aluminum foil on a flat surface.
2. In a small bowl, mash the avocado with a fork.
3. Spread half of the avocado mixture on the nori sheet, leaving a 1/2-inch strip uncovered along the top edge. Sprinkle 1 tablespoon of the sesame seeds (if using), evenly over the avocado. Arrange 2 pieces of the smoked salmon horizontally, covering the avocado.
4. Arrange the cucumber horizontally, running up the length of the sheet and creating columns to cover the salmon.
5. Wet the tip of your finger and run it along the exposed seam. Roll the nori tightly away from you, using the foil as a guide and pressing firmly to seal. Repeat the process with the remaining nori sheet and ingredients, and refrigerate both for at least 30 minutes to firm up.
6. Using a very sharp or serrated knife, slice each roll into 6 to 8 pieces. Serve with pickled ginger and wasabi (if using) and soy sauce for dipping.

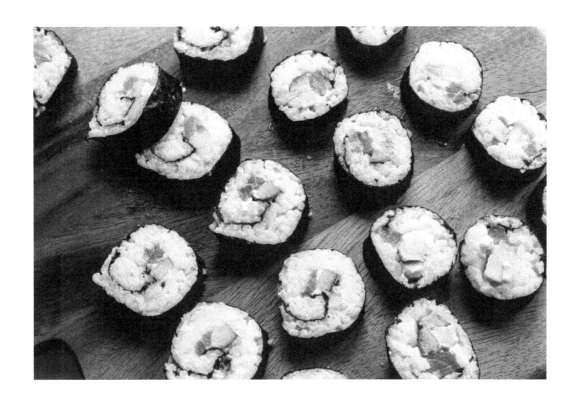

Nutrition:

Calories: 457

Carbs: 45.2g

Fat: 18.6g

Fiber: 2.8g

Protein: 25.7g

24. Oil-Poached Whitefish with Lemony Gremolata

Preparation time: 10 minutes

Cooking time: 15 minutes

Servings: 4

Ingredients:

- 2 3/4pound skinless Arctic char or other whitefish fillets
- 1 teaspoon kosher salt
- 1 teaspoon freshly ground black pepper
- 1/2 cup extra-virgin olive oil
- 3 cloves garlic, minced
- 3/4 cup fresh parsley leaves, minced, divided
- 1/4 cup grated lemon zest (from 6 small or 4 large lemons), divided

Directions:

1. Place the fish fillets lengthwise in a 13-by-9-inch baking dish and season with the salt and pepper on both sides. In a small bowl, whisk together the olive oil, garlic, half of the parsley, and half of the lemon zest. Pour evenly over the fish, cover, and marinate in the refrigerator for at least 30 minutes and up to overnight.
2. Preheat the oven to 350F.
3. Bake the fish until just cooked through, 15 to 20 minutes. Cut each fillet into 2 pieces, top evenly with the remaining parsley and lemon zest, and serve with Lemony Sautéed Chard with Red Onion and Herbs or another vegetable side or salad.

Nutrition:

Calories: 620   Carbs: 89g

Fat: 22g   Fiber: 12g

Protein: 18g

25. Ceviche Fish Tacos with Easy Guacamole

Preparation time: 10 minutes

Cooking time: 6 hours minutes

Servings: 2

Ingredients:

Ceviche:

- 11/4 pounds meaty skinless fresh fish fillets
- 3 tablespoons lime juice
- 3 tablespoons lemon juice
- 1/4 teaspoon salt
- 1/4 teaspoon freshly ground black pepper
- 2 ripe plum or heirloom tomatoes, seeded and chopped (juices reserved)
- 1 tablespoon olive oil
- 3/4 cup chopped red onion
- 1 serrano pepper, seeded and minced (optional)
- Bibb lettuce leaves, for serving

Guacamole:

- 4 avocados
- Juice from 1/2 lime (reserve remaining half for wedges, for serving)
- 1/2 cup chopped fresh cilantro
- 2 tablespoons chopped red onion
- 1 serrano pepper, seeded and minced

Additional Taco Fixings:

- Store-bought salsa (without added salt, oil, or sugar)
- Creamy Citrus Slaw
- Chopped fresh cilantro
- Lime wedges
- Quick-Pickled Red Onions

Directions:

1. In a medium bowl, place the fish, lime and lemon juices, salt, and pepper and toss to combine. Cover tightly and chill until the fish turns completely white, tossing occasionally, at least 4 hours and up to 6 hours.
2. Meanwhile, make the guacamole. Cut the avocados in half, then remove the pit and peel. Spoon the avocado into a large bowl and mash it with a large metal spoon. Add the lime juice and continue to mix and mash until mostly smooth with some remaining chunks (this helps prevent the guacamole from browning). Mix in the cilantro, onion, and serrano pepper. Cover tightly and refrigerate until ready to use.
3. Strain the fish, moving it to a clean bowl; discard the marinade. Add the tomatoes, oil, onion, and serrano pepper (if using) and toss gently to combine. Serve wrapped in the Bibb lettuce leaves topped with the guacamole and your choice of additional fixings.

Nutrition:

Calories: 253

Carbs: 107g

Fat: 5g

Fiber: 36g

Protein: 32g

26. Shrimp Scampi with Baby Spinach

Preparation time: 10 minutes

Cooking time: 10 minutes

Servings: 2-4

Ingredients:

- 1 pound jumbo shrimp (about 12), peeled and deveined
- 3 tablespoons extra-virgin olive oil, divided
- 6 cloves garlic, minced
- 1 cup unsalted chicken broth or stock
- Grated zest and juice from 1 medium lemon
- 1/2 teaspoon red pepper flakes, or to taste
- 1/4 teaspoon sea salt or Himalayan salt, or to taste
- 1/2 teaspoon freshly ground black pepper, or to taste
- 1/4 cup 1/2 stick) cold unsalted grass-fed butter, cubed
- 6 to 8 cups (6 ounces) baby spinach leaves
- 2 to 3 tablespoons chopped fresh parsley (optional)

Directions:

1. Pat the shrimp very dry with paper towels. Heat 2 tablespoons of the olive oil in a large skillet over medium-high heat. Add the shrimp and cook until pink, flipping once, about 2 minutes per side. Transfer to a large bowl or plate.
2. Reduce the heat to medium and add remaining 1 tablespoon oil. Add the garlic and cook until just fragrant, about 1 minute. Add the broth, lemon zest and juice, red pepper flakes, salt, and black pepper, increase the heat to medium-high, and bring to a simmer. Reduce the sauce by half, scraping up any browned bits from the bottom with a wooden spoon, about 5 minutes.
3. Remove the pan from the heat and allow to cool slightly. Add butter, one cube at a time, stirring continually with a wooden spoon until the sauce thickens.
4. To serve, divide spinach evenly among four plates. Top each plate with about 4 shrimp. Divide the sauce evenly among the plates and garnish with the parsley (if using).

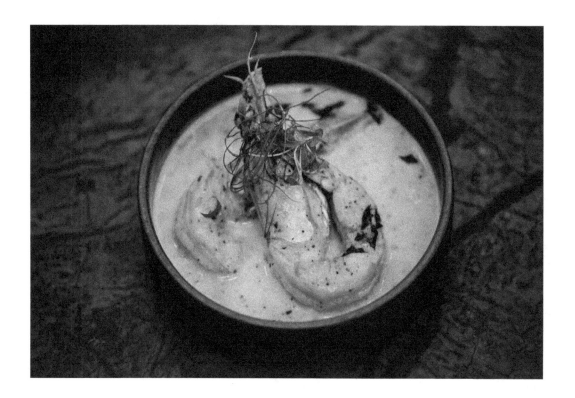

Nutrition:

Calories: 268   Carbs: 40g

Fat: 7.4g   Fiber: 3.5g

Protein: 11g

27. Shrimp Fried Rice

Preparation time: 10 minutes

Cooking time: 25 minutes

Servings: 4

Ingredients:

- 3 tablespoons gluten-free soy sauce, tamari, or coconut aminos
- 2 tablespoons minced fresh ginger
- 3 tablespoons sesame oil, divided
- 2 large eggs, lightly beaten
- 2/3 to 3/4 pound medium shrimp, peeled and deveined (about 24)
- 1 shallot, minced
- 1 red bell pepper, seeded and diced
- 1 recipe cooled or chilled Easy Cauliflower Rice
- 3/4 cup frozen peas
- 1/4 cup chopped unsalted cashews
- 2 tablespoons chopped fresh cilantro
- 1/4 teaspoon red pepper flakes (optional)
- Sliced scallion greens, for garnish (optional)

Directions:

1. In a small bowl, whisk the soy sauce and ginger together and set aside.
2. In a wok or large skillet over medium heat, heat 1 tablespoon of the sesame oil. Add the eggs and cook, stirring frequently with a wooden spoon or spatula, until scrambled. Transfer to a small bowl and break up the cooked egg into small pieces using two forks. Set aside.
3. In the same wok over medium-high heat, heat 1 tablespoon of the sesame oil. Add the shrimp and cook, tossing, until bright pink but not browned, 3 to 4 minutes. Transfer the shrimp to a separate plate or bowl and set aside.
4. Add the remaining 1 tablespoon sesame oil and the shallot to the wok and cook until fragrant, tossing frequently, about 30 seconds. Add the bell pepper and cook until just

tender, tossing occasionally, about 2 minutes. Add the cauliflower rice and cook, tossing occasionally, until lightly browned and crisp, about 5 minutes. Stir in the soy sauce mixture. Add the cooked shrimp, cooked eggs, and peas and stir until well combined and heated through, 2 to 3 minutes. Add the cashews, cilantro, and red pepper flakes (if using), tossing to combine.

5. Divide the mixture among four bowls, garnish with scallion greens (if using) and serve.

Nutrition:

Calories: 116   Carbs: 24g

Fat: 1g   Fiber: 4g

Protein: 4g

28. Mussels with Lemon-Garlic-Herb Broth

Preparation time: 10 minutes

Cooking time: 8 minutes

Servings: 4

Ingredients:

- 2 pounds mussels
- 1 tablespoon extra-virgin olive oil
- 2 shallots, minced
- 3 cloves garlic, minced
- 2 cups chicken or Veggie Trimmings Stock
- 1/4 cup lemon juice (from 2 lemons)
- 1/4 cup chopped fresh parsley, plus more for garnish
- 1/4 cup chopped fresh dill (optional)
- 3 tablespoons chopped fresh thyme
- 1/2 teaspoon salt
- 1/4 teaspoon freshly ground black pepper
- 1/4 teaspoon red pepper flakes (optional)
- 3 cups baby spinach (or spinach leaves torn into smaller pieces)
- 2 tablespoons cold unsalted grass-fed butter, cubed

Directions:

1. Rinse the mussels under cold running water, pulling off their black beards as needed. Place in a strainer to drain and set aside.
2. Heat the oil in a large, deep skillet, stockpot, or Dutch oven over medium-high heat. Add the shallots and cook, stirring, until soft and translucent, about 2 minutes. Add the garlic and cook until fragrant, 30 seconds. Add the stock, lemon juice, herbs, salt, pepper, and red pepper flakes (if using), and stirring to combine. Bring the stock to a boil.

3. Add the mussels, cover, and cook, undisturbed, until the mussels open their shells, about 5 minutes. Reduce the heat to low. Discard any mussels that have not yet opened. Divide the mussels among four large serving bowls.

4. Add the spinach to the broth, cover, and cook until just wilted, 1 to 2 minutes. Remove the lid and turn off the heat. Let sit for 1 minute, then add the cold butter, one piece at a time, stirring in each one until fully melted before adding the next one.

5. Spoon the broth over the mussels in the bowls, garnish with more parsley if you like, and serve.

Nutrition:

Calories: 194   Carbs: 33g

Fat: 3g   Fiber: 8g

Protein: 10g

29. Clam Linguine with Zucchini Noodles

Preparation time: 10 minutes

Cooking time: 20 minutes

Servings: 4

Ingredients:

- 2 medium zucchini
- 2 tablespoons extra-virgin olive oil
- 4 cloves garlic, minced
- 4 (6-ounce) cans chopped clams
- 1/2 teaspoon red pepper flakes
- 1/4 cup 1/2 stick) cold unsalted grass-fed butter, cubed
- 2 teaspoons grated lemon zest
- Chopped fresh parsley, for garnish
- Freshly ground black pepper
- 2 lemon wedges, for garnish (optional)

Directions:

1. Using a paralyzer, cut the zucchini into noodles or use purchased zoodles (thaw if frozen). Set aside.
2. In a large, deep skillet over medium-high heat, heat olive oil and garlic until fragrant, 1 to 2 minutes, taking care that the garlic doesn't brown. Drain the liquid from clams into the skillet, leaving the clams in the cans. Add the red pepper flakes. Bring to a simmer and cook until the liquid is reduced to 3/4 cup, about 15 minutes.
3. Add the clams to the broth and cook until heated through, about 1 minute. Turn off the heat and let sit for 1 minute.
4. Add the butter, stirring in each cube until fully melted before adding the next one. Stir in the lemon zest. Add zucchini noodles and toss to coat.
5. To serve, divide between four plates or shallow bowls. Top with parsley and black pepper, and serve with lemon wedges, if desired.

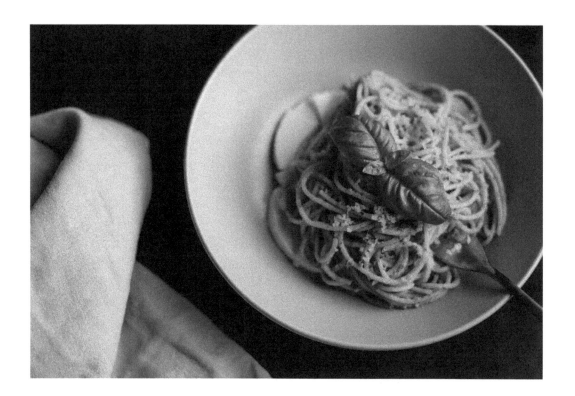

Nutrition:

Calories: 250   Carbs: 13g

Fat: 20g   Fiber: 2g

Protein: 6g

30. Crab Cakes with Creamy Citrus Slaw

Preparation time: 10 minutes

Cooking time: 7 minutes

Servings: 2

Ingredients:

- 1 (14-ounce) package shredded coleslaw mix
- Grated zest and juice of 1 medium lemon
- Grated zest of 1 medium navel orange
- 2 tablespoons Dijon mustard

Crab Cakes:

- 2 large eggs
- 1 tablespoon Dijon mustard
- 1/2 teaspoon sea salt
- 1/2 teaspoon Old Bay seasoning or paprika
- 1/4 teaspoon freshly ground black pepper
- 1 (16-ounce) can cooked jumbo lump crab meat, drained and patted dry
- 3/4 cup cooled or chilled cooked Easy Cauliflower Rice, mashed with a fork
- 2 tablespoons chopped fresh parsley
- 2 tablespoons extra-virgin olive oil

Directions:

1. To make the slaw, toss the coleslaw mix with the lemon zest and juice, orange zest, and mustard in a large bowl until evenly coated. Refrigerate for at least 30 minutes.
2. In a medium bowl, whisk together the eggs, mustard, salt, Old Bay seasoning, and pepper. Fold in the crab, cauliflower rice, and parsley until well combined. Refrigerate until slightly firm, about 10 minutes.
3. Remove the crab mixture from the refrigerator and form into four patties about 2 inches thick and 3 inches in diameter.

4. Heat the olive oil in a large skillet or cast iron pan over medium-high heat. When the oil is hot, add two of the crab cakes. Cook until golden brown, about 3 minutes per side. Transfer to a paper towel–lined plate. Repeat with the remaining cakes.

5. Place two crab cakes on each plate and serve with the chilled slaw.

Nutrition:

Calories: 230   Carbs: 41g

Fat: 4g   Fiber: 10g

Protein: 11g

31. Peppery Shrimp and Steak for Two

Preparation time: 10 minutes

Cooking time: 25 minutes

Servings: 2

Ingredients:

- 12 medium shrimp, peeled and deveined
- 2 filet mignon steaks
- 2 Teaspoons olive oil
- 1 Tablespoon butter, melted
- 1 Tablespoon finely minced onion
- 1 Teaspoon steak seasoning
- 1 Tablespoon finely minced onion
- 1 Tablespoon white wine
- 1 Teaspoon Worcestershire sauce
- 1 Teaspoon seafood seasoning
- 1/8 Teaspoon freshly ground black pepper
- 1 Teaspoon lemon juice
- 1 Teaspoon dried parsley

Directions:

1. In a bowl, whisk 1 Tablespoon olive oil, onion, butter, Worcestershire sauce, wine, lemon juice, parsley, seafood seasoning, garlic, and black pepper together
2. Toss to coat evenly. Cover bowl with plastic wrap and refrigerate for flavors to blend, at least 15 minutes.
3. Preheat an outdoor grill for medium-high heat and lightly oil the grate. Coat steaks with 2 Teaspoons olive oil; sprinkle with steak seasoning.
4. Cook steaks until they are beginning to firm and have reached your desired doneness, 5 to 7 minutes per side.
5. Transfer steaks to a platter and loosely tent with a piece of aluminum foil.

6. Remove shrimp from marinade and grill until they are bright pink on the outside and the meat is no longer transparent in the canter, 2 to 3 minutes per side.

Nutrition:

Calories: 226

Carbs: 41g

Fat: 5g

Fiber: 7g

Protein: 7g

32. Creamy Salmon Capers with Spiralled Zoodles

Preparation time: 10 minutes

Cooking time: 5 minutes

Servings: 2

Ingredients:

- A small shallot, chopped
- 1 Tablespoon of almond flour
- 1 cup sour cream
- 1/2 cup parmesan
- 1/3 cup sliced mushrooms of your choice
- 1 cup broccoli florets
- 1 Tablespoon capers
- 1 Tablespoon chopped chives
- 2 tablespoons s chopped parsley
- 2 fillets of wild Alaskan salmon
- 1 Tablespoon avocado oil
- 3 Tablespoon s pastured butter
- 2 cloves of garlic, minced
- Lemon juice to taste
- Black pepper to taste

Directions:

1. Descale and wash the fish. Fry the salmon with the avocado oil for a few minutes, turning once (do not overcook).
2. Remove its skin and eat it. Add lemon juice on the fish, and set aside.
3. Heat water in a small water and add the mushrooms to boil for a few minutes.
4. Add the broccoli florets for another 1-2 minutes (must remain a little bit crunchy). Strain, set aside.
5. In a large pot heat the butter with the black pepper, garlic and shallot.

6. Add the sour cream and parmesan when browned. Stir to combine, but don't let it get too cooked (no more than 30 seconds on fire, just enough for the parmesan to melt).
7. Cut the salmon in small pieces, add it to the cream.
8. Add the mushrooms, broccoli, and capers, and carefully combine.
9. Sprinkle with chives or parsley; serve with spiralled "zoodles".

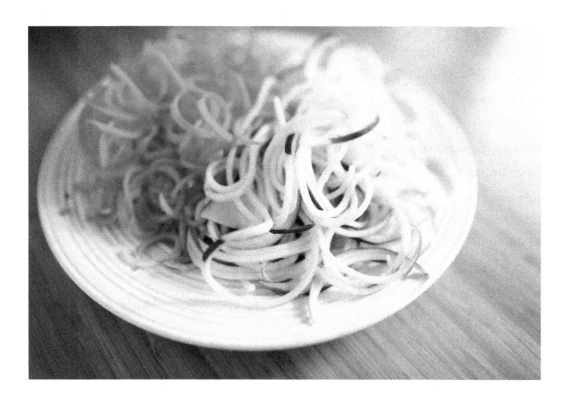

Nutrition:

Calories: 135

Carbs: 11g

Fat: 9.8g

Fiber: 4g

Protein: 3.9g

33. Garlicky Fish Fillets with Parsley leaves

Preparation time: 10 minutes

Cooking time: 30 minutes

Servings: 4

Ingredients:

- 2 skinless Arctic char or other whitefish fillets
- 1 Teaspoon kosher salt
- 1 Teaspoon freshly ground black pepper
- 1/2 cup extra-virgin olive oil
- 3 cloves garlic, minced
- 3/4 cup fresh parsley leaves, minced, divided
- 1/4 cup grated lemon zest (from 6 small or 4 large lemons), divided

Directions:

1. Place the fish fillets lengthwise in a 13-by-9-inch baking dish and season with the salt and pepper on both sides.
2. In a small bowl, whisk together the olive oil, garlic, half of the parsley, and half of the lemon zest. Pour evenly over the fish, cover, and marinate in the refrigerator for at least 30 minutes and up to overnight.
3. Preheat the oven to 350F. 3. Bake the fish until just cooked through, 15 to 20 minutes.
4. Cut each fillet into 2 pieces, top evenly with the remaining parsley and lemon zest, and serve with Lemony Sautéed Chard with Red Onion and Herbs or another vegetable side or salad.

Nutrition:

Calories: 279.4   Carbs: 45.8 g

Fat: 8 g   Fiber: 5 g

Protein: 10.5 g

34. Easy Butter Shrimp Scampi with Parsley Leaves

Preparation time: 10 minutes

Cooking time: 10 minutes

Servings: 3

Ingredients:

- 454 g jumbo shrimp (about 12), peeled and deveined
- 3 Tablespoons extra-virgin olive oil, divided
- 6 cloves garlic, minced
- 1 cup unsalted chicken broth or stock
- Grated zest and juice from
- 1 medium lemon
- 1/2 Teaspoon red pepper flakes, or to taste
- 1/4 Teaspoon sea salt or Himalayan salt, or to taste
- 1/2 Teaspoon freshly ground black pepper, or to taste
- 1/4 cup (1/2 stick) cold unsalted grass-fed butter, cubed
- 8 cups baby spinach leaves
- 2 to 3 Tablespoons chopped fresh parsley (optional)

Directions:

1. Pat the shrimp very dry with paper towels. Heat 2 tablespoons of the olive oil in a large skillet over medium-high heat.
2. Add the shrimp and cook until pink, flipping once, about 2 minutes per side. Transfer to a large bowl or plate. 2
3. Reduce the heat to medium and add remaining 1 Tablespoon oil. Add the garlic and cook until just fragrant, about 1 minute.
4. Add the broth, lemon zest and juice, red pepper flakes, salt, and black pepper, increase the heat to medium-high, and bring to a simmer.
5. Reduce the sauce by half, scraping up any browned bits from the bottom with a wooden spoon, about 5 minutes.

6. Remove the pan from the heat and allow cooling slightly. Add butter, one cube at a time, stirring continually with a wooden spoon until the sauce thickens.
7. To serve, divide spinach evenly among four plates. Top each plate with about 4 shrimp. Divide the sauce evenly among the plates and garnish with the parsley.

Nutrition:

Calories: 147

Carbs: 21.2g

Fat: 5g

Fiber: 1.5g

Protein: 3.8g

35. One pan Broiled Salmon with Yellow Miso

Preparation time: 10 minutes

Cooking time: 10 minutes

Servings: 2

Ingredients:

- 2 salmon fillets
- 1/4 cup white or yellow miso
- 2 tablespoons rice or coconut vinegar
- 2 tablespoons sesame oil, divided
- 1 Tablespoon gluten-free soy sauce, tamari, or coconut amino
- 1 Tablespoon minced fresh ginger
- 1 clove garlic, minced
- 680 g (medium bunch) baby bok choy, core removed, sliced into 11/2-inch pieces, white stem and leafy green parts separated
- 2 tablespoons thinly sliced scallion whites (optional)
- 2 tablespoons thinly sliced scallion greens, for garnish (optional)

Directions:

1. Heat the broiler to high.
2. On a baking sheet or broiler pan, place the salmon, skin-side down, and pat it dry.
3. In a small bowl, whisk together the miso, vinegar, 1 Tablespoon of the sesame oil, the soy sauce, ginger, and garlic.
4. Spread 2 tablespoons of the glaze evenly over the top of the salmon, setting aside the remainder. Let it stand for 10 minutes, if you have time.
5. Broil the salmon until the glaze is bubbly, 3 to 4 minutes. Cover it loosely with foil and continue to broil until slightly pink in the center, another 3 to 4 minutes.
6. Remove the salmon from the broiler, remove the foil, and let it cool.
7. In a large skillet over medium-high heat, heat the remaining 1 Tablespoon sesame oil.

8. Add the bok choy stems and scallion whites (if using) and cook until just tender, 2 to 3 minutes.
9. Stir in the remaining miso glaze and cook until fragrant, 30 to 60 seconds.
10. Add the bok choy greens, cover, and steam until just wilted, 30 seconds. Toss to coat with the sauce.
11. To serve, divide the bok choy evenly between two plates.
12. Top each with a salmon fillet and sprinkle with scallion greens (if using).

Nutrition:

Calories: 191

Carbs: 22g

Fat: 10g

Fiber: 3.3g

Protein: 4.1g

36. Garlic and Herb Mussels in Rose Broth

Preparation time: 10 minutes

Cooking time: 10 minutes

Servings: 4

Ingredients:

- 32 ounce mussels
- 1 Tablespoon extra-virgin olive oil
- 2 shallots, minced
- 3 cloves garlic, minced
- 2 cups chicken or Veggie Trimmings Stock
- 1/4 cup lemon juice (from 2 lemons)
- 1/4 cup chopped fresh parsley, plus more for garnish
- 1/4 cup chopped fresh dill (optional)
- 3 Tablespoons chopped fresh thyme
- 1/2 Teaspoon salt
- 1/4 Teaspoon freshly ground black pepper
- 1/4 Teaspoon red pepper flakes (optional)
- 3 cups baby spinach (or spinach leaves torn into smaller pieces)
- 2 tablespoons cold unsalted grass-fed butter, cubed

Directions:

1. Rinse the mussels under cold running water, pulling off their black beards as needed. Place in a strainer to drain and set aside.
2. Heat the oil in a large, deep skillet, stockpot, or Dutch oven over medium-high heat.
3. Add the shallots and cook, stirring, until soft and translucent, about 2 minutes. Add the garlic and cook until fragrant, 30 seconds.
4. Add the stock, lemon juice, herbs, salt, pepper, and red pepper flakes (if using), and stirring to combine. Bring the stock to a boil.

5. Add the mussels, cover, and cook, undisturbed, until the mussels open their shells, about 5 minutes.
6. Reduce the heat to low. Discard any mussels that have not yet opened. Divide the mussels among four large serving bowls.
7. Add the spinach to the broth, cover, and cook until just wilted, 1 to 2 minutes. Remove the lid and turn off the heat. Let sit for 1 minute, then add the cold butter, one piece at a time, stirring in each one until fully melted before adding the next one.
8. Spoon the broth over the mussels in the bowls, garnish with more parsley if you like, and serve.

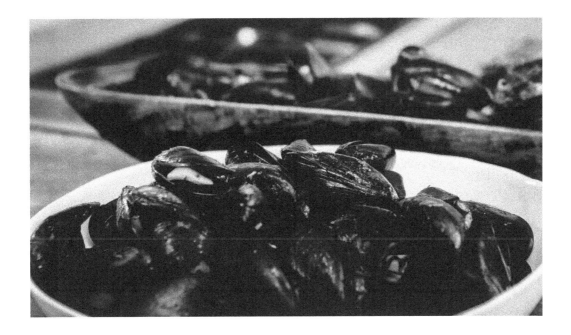

Nutrition:

Calories: 192   Carbs: 14.3g

Fat: 9.7g   Fiber: 5.2g

Protein: 11.4g

37. Spicy Crabs with Chilled Coleslaw Mix

Preparation time: 10 minutes

Cooking time: 30 minutes

Servings: 2

Ingredients:

- 1 package shredded coleslaw mix
- Grated zest and juice of 1 medium lemon
- Grated zest of 1 medium navel orange
- 2 tablespoons Dijon mustard
- 2 large eggs
- 1 Tablespoon Dijon mustard
- 1/2 Teaspoon sea salt
- 1/2 Teaspoon Old Bay seasoning or paprika
- 1/4 Teaspoon freshly ground black pepper
- 1 can cooked jumbo lump crab meat, drained and patted dry
- 3/4 cup cooled or chilled cooked
- Easy Cauliflower Rice, mashed with a fork
- 2 tablespoons chopped fresh parsley
- 2 tablespoons extra-virgin olive oil

Directions:

1. To make the slaw, toss the coleslaw mix with the lemon zest and juice, orange zest, and mustard in a large bowl until evenly coated.
2. Refrigerate it for at least 30 minutes.
3. In a medium bowl, whisk together the eggs, mustard, salt, Old Bay seasoning, and pepper.
4. Fold in the crab, cauliflower rice, and parsley until well combined. Refrigerate until slightly firm, about 10 minutes.
5. Remove the crab mixture from the refrigerator and form into four patties about 2 inches thick and 3 inches in diameter.

6. Heat the olive oil in a large skillet or cast-iron pan over medium-high heat. When the oil is hot, add two of the crab cakes.
7. Cook until golden brown, about 3 minutes per side. Transfer to a paper towel–lined plate. Repeat with the remaining cakes.
8. Place two crab cakes on each plate and serve with the chilled slaw.

Nutrition:

Calories: 265

Carbs: 19.8g

Fat: 18.4g

Fiber: 8.1g

Protein: 4.6g

38. Coconut Salmon with Scallion Greens

Preparation time: 10 minutes

Cooking time: 15 minutes

Servings: 2

Ingredients:

- 2 (6-ounce) salmon fillets
- 1/4 cup white or yellow miso
- 2 tablespoons rice or coconut vinegar
- 2 tablespoons sesame oil, divided
- 1 tablespoon gluten-free soy sauce, tamari, or coconut amino
- 1 tablespoon minced fresh ginger
- 1 clove garlic, minced
- 11/2 pounds (medium bunch) baby bok choy, core removed, sliced into 11/2-inch pieces, white stem and leafy green parts separated
- 2 tablespoons thinly sliced scallion whites (optional)
- 2 tablespoons thinly sliced scallion greens, for garnish (optional)

Directions:

1. Heat the broiler to high.
2. On a baking sheet or broiler pan, place the salmon, skin-side down, and pat it dry.
3. In a small bowl, whisk together the miso, vinegar, 1 tablespoon of the sesame oil, the soy sauce, ginger, and garlic.
4. Spread 2 tablespoons of the glaze evenly over the top of the salmon, setting aside the remainder. Let it stand for 10 minutes, if you have time.
5. Broil the salmon until the glaze is bubbly, 3 to 4 minutes.
6. Cover it loosely with foil and continue to broil until slightly pink in the center, another 3 to 4 minutes.
7. Remove the salmon from the broiler, remove the foil, and let it cool.
8. In a large skillet over medium-high heat, heat the remaining 1 tablespoon sesame oil.

9. Add the bok choy stems and scallion whites (if using) and cook until just tender, 2 to 3 minutes.

10. Stir in the remaining miso glaze and cook until fragrant, 30 to 60 seconds.

11. Add the bok choy greens, cover, and steam until just wilted, 30 seconds. Toss to coat with the sauce.

12. To serve, divide the bok choy evenly between two plates. Top each with a salmon fillet and sprinkle with scallion greens (if using).

Nutrition:

Calories: 291   Carbs: 37.2g

Fat: 12.4g   Fiber: 2.3g

Protein: 6.4g

39. Soy dipped Avocado Sushi Roll

Preparation time: 10 minutes

Cooking time: 0 minutes

Servings: 2

Ingredients:

- 2 sheets sushi nori
- 1 medium avocado, pitted and peeled
- 2 tablespoons sesame seeds, divided (optional)
- 4 ounces smoked salmon (about 4 thin slices)
- 1 medium cucumber, cut into matchsticks
- 3 tablespoons pickled ginger (optional)
- 1 teaspoon wasabi paste (optional)
- Gluten-free soy sauce, tamari, or coconut amino, for dipping

Directions:

1. Lay 1 piece of nori on a sheet of parchment paper or aluminium foil on a flat surface.
2. In a small bowl, mash the avocado with a fork.
3. Spread half of the avocado mixture on the nori sheet, leaving a 1/2-inch strip uncovered along the top edge.
4. Sprinkle 1 tablespoon of the sesame seeds (if using), evenly over the avocado. Arrange 2 pieces of the smoked salmon horizontally, covering the avocado.
5. Arrange the cucumber horizontally, running up the length of the sheet and creating columns to cover the salmon.
6. Wet the tip of your finger and run it along the exposed seam. Roll the nori tightly away from you, using the foil as a guide and pressing firmly to seal.
7. Repeat the process with the remaining nori sheet and ingredients, and refrigerate both for at least 30 minutes to firm up.
8. Using a very sharp or serrated knife, slice each roll into 6 to 8 pieces. Serve with pickled ginger and wasabi and soy sauce for dipping

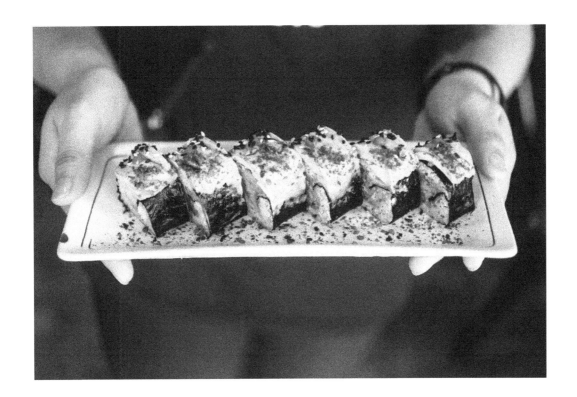

Nutrition:

Calories: 115   Carbs: 5.3g

Fat: 8.5g   Fiber: 2.6g

Protein: 3.3g

40. Baked Garlic marinade Arctic char Fillets

Preparation time: 10 minutes

Cooking time: 30 minutes

Servings: 4

Ingredients:

- 2 3/4pound skinless Arctic char or other whitefish fillets
- 1 teaspoon kosher salt
- 1 teaspoon freshly ground black pepper
- 1/2 cup extra-virgin olive oil
- 3 cloves garlic, minced
- 3/4 cup fresh parsley leaves, minced, divided
- 1/4 cup grated lemon zest (from 6 small or 4 large lemons), divided

Directions:

1. Place the fish fillets lengthwise in a 13-by-9-inch baking dish and season with the salt and pepper on both sides.
2. In a small bowl, whisk together the olive oil, garlic, half of the parsley, and half of the lemon zest.
3. Pour evenly over the fish, cover, and marinate in the refrigerator for at least 30 minutes and up to overnight.
4. Preheat the oven to 350F.
5. Bake the fish until just cooked through, 15 to 20 minutes.
6. Cut each fillet into 2 pieces, top evenly with the remaining parsley and lemon zest and serve.

Nutrition:

Calories: 123

Carbs: 13.6g

Fat: 7g

Fiber: 2g

Protein: 1.2g

41. Spicy Cilantro Fish wrapped in Lettuce Leaves

Preparation time: 10 minutes

Cooking time: 20 minutes

Servings: 4

Ingredients:

- 11/4 pounds meaty skinless fresh fish fillets (wild-caught or Hamachi tuna, halibut, tilapia, barramundi, or mahi mahi), cut into 1/2-inch cubes
- 3 tablespoons lime juice
- 3 tablespoons lemon juice
- 1/4 teaspoon salt
- 1/4 teaspoons freshly ground black pepper
- 2 ripe plum or heirloom tomatoes, seeded and chopped (juices reserved)
- 1 tablespoon olive oil
- 3/4 cup chopped red onion
- 1 Serrano pepper, seeded and minced (optional)
- Bibb lettuce leaves, for serving
- 4 avocados
- Juice from 1/2 lime (reserve remaining half for wedges, for serving)
- 1/2 cup chopped fresh cilantro
- 2 tablespoons chopped red onion
- 1 Serrano pepper, seeded and minced
- Chopped fresh cilantro
- Lime wedges

Directions:

1. In a medium bowl, place the fish, lime and lemon juices, salt, and pepper and toss to combine.
2. Cover tightly and chill until the fish turns completely white, tossing occasionally, at least 4 hours and up to 6 hours.

3. Meanwhile, make the guacamole. Cut the avocados in half, and then remove the pit and peel.
4. Spoon the avocado into a large bowl and mash it with a large metal spoon.
5. Add the lime juice and continue to mix and mash until mostly smooth with some remaining chunks (this helps prevent the guacamole from browning).
6. Mix in the cilantro, onion, and Serrano pepper. Cover tightly and refrigerate until ready to use.
7. Strain the fish, moving it to a clean bowl; discard the marinade. Add the tomatoes, oil, onion, and Serrano pepper (if using) and toss gently to combine.
8. Serve wrapped in the lettuce leaves topped with the guacamole and your choice of additional fixings.

Nutrition:

Calories: 203   Carbs: 5.1g

Fat: 19.6g   Fiber: 4.6g

Protein: 1.5g

42. Homemade Shrimp and Pea Bowl with Cashews

Preparation time: 10 minutes

Cooking time: 20 minutes

Servings: 4

Ingredients:

- 3 tablespoons gluten-free soy sauce, tamari, or coconut amino
- 2 tablespoons minced fresh ginger
- 3 tablespoons sesame oil, divided
- 2 large eggs, lightly beaten
- 2/3 to 3/4 pound medium shrimp, peeled and deveined (about 24)
- 1 shallot, minced
- 1 red bell pepper, seeded and diced
- 3/4 cup frozen peas
- 1/4 cup chopped unsalted cashews
- 2 tablespoons chopped fresh cilantro
- 1/4 teaspoon red pepper flakes (optional)
- Sliced scallion greens, for garnish (optional)

Directions:

1. In a small bowl, whisk the soy sauce and ginger together and set aside.
2. In a wok or large skillet over medium heat, heat 1 tablespoon of the sesame oil.
3. Add the eggs and cook, stirring frequently with a wooden spoon or spatula, until scrambled.
4. Transfer to a small bowl and break up the cooked egg into small pieces using two forks. Set aside.
5. In the same wok over medium-high heat, heat 1 tablespoon of the sesame oil.
6. Add the shrimp and cook, tossing, until bright pink but not browned, 3 to 4 minutes.
7. Transfer the shrimp to a separate plate or bowl and set aside.

8. Add the remaining 1 tablespoon sesame oil and the shallot to the wok and cook until fragrant, tossing frequently, about 30 seconds.
9. Add the bell pepper and cook until just tender, tossing occasionally, about 2 minutes.
10. Add the cauliflower rice and cook, tossing occasionally, until lightly browned and crisp, about 5 minutes.
11. Stir in the soy sauce mixture. Add the cooked shrimp, cooked eggs, and peas and stir until well combined and heated through, 2 to 3 minutes.
12. Add the cashews, cilantro, and red pepper flakes (if using), tossing to combine.
13. Divide the mixture among four bowls, garnish with scallion greens (if using) and serve.

Nutrition:

Calories: 108

Carbs: 3.2g

Fat: 9.8g

Fiber: 1.8g

Protein: 1.1g

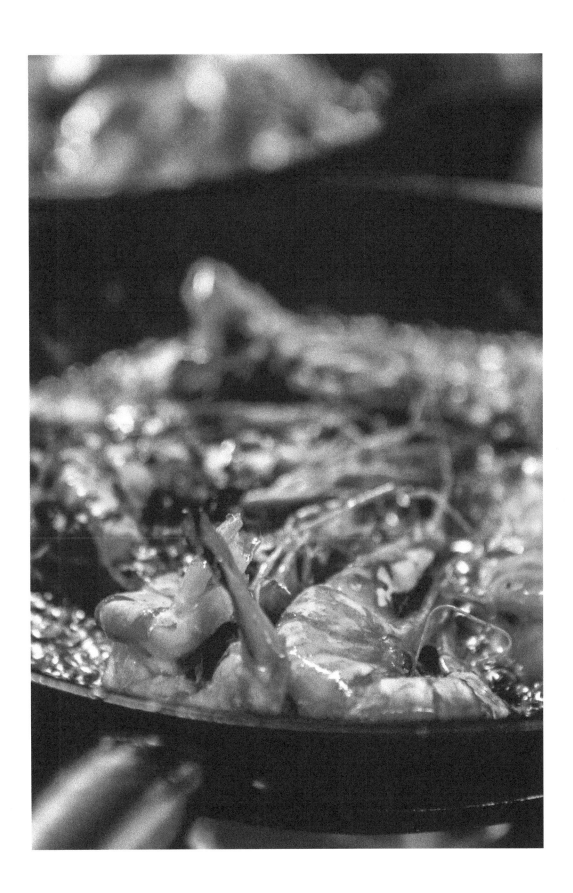

43. Mussel Spinach Cold Butter Bowl

Preparation time: 10 minutes

Cooking time: 8 minutes

Servings: 4

Ingredients:

- 2 pounds mussels
- 1 tablespoon extra-virgin olive oil
- 2 shallots, minced
- 3 cloves garlic, minced
- 1/4 cup lemon juice (from 2 lemons)
- 1/4 cup chopped fresh parsley, plus more for garnish
- 1/4 cup chopped fresh dill (optional)
- 3 tablespoons chopped fresh thyme
- 1/2 teaspoon salt
- 1/4 teaspoons freshly ground black pepper
- 1/4 teaspoon red pepper flakes (optional)
- 3 cups baby spinach (or spinach leaves torn into smaller pieces)
- 2 tablespoons cold unsalted grass-fed butter, cubed

Directions:

1. Rinse the mussels under cold running water, pulling off their black beards as needed. Place in a strainer to drain and set aside.
2. Heat the oil in a large, deep skillet, stockpot, or Dutch oven over medium-high heat.
3. Add the shallots and cook, stirring, until soft and translucent, about 2 minutes.
4. Add the garlic and cook until fragrant, 30 seconds. Add the stock, lemon juice, herbs, salt, pepper, and red pepper flakes (if using), and stirring to combine. Bring the stock to a boil.
5. Add the mussels, cover, and cook, undisturbed, until the mussels open their shells, about 5 minutes.

6. Reduce the heat to low. Discard any mussels that have not yet opened. Divide the mussels among four large serving bowls.

7. Add the spinach to the broth, cover, and cook until just wilted, 1 to 2 minutes. Remove the lid and turn off the heat. Let sit for 1 minute, then add the cold butter, one piece at a time, stirring in each one until fully melted before adding the next one.

8. Spoon the broth over the mussels in the bowls, garnish with more parsley if you like, and serve.

Nutrition:

Calories: 299   Carbs: 48.5g

Fat: 7.6g   Fiber: 5.4g

Protein: 9g

44. Creamy Zucchini Clam Shallow Bowls

Preparation time: 10 minutes

Cooking time: 20 minutes

Servings: 4

Ingredients:

- 2 medium zucchini
- 2 tablespoons extra-virgin olive oil
- 4 cloves garlic, minced
- 4 (6-ounce) cans chopped clams
- 1/2 teaspoon red pepper flakes
- 1/4 cup 1/2 stick cold unsalted grass-fed butter, cubed
- 2 teaspoons grated lemon zest
- Chopped fresh parsley, for garnish
- Freshly ground black pepper
- 2 lemon wedges, for garnish (optional)

Directions:

1. Using a spiralized, cut the zucchini into noodles or use purchased zoodles (thaw if frozen). Set aside.
2. In a large, deep skillet over medium-high heat, heat olive oil and garlic until fragrant, 1 to 2 minutes, taking care that the garlic doesn't brown.
3. Drain the liquid from clams into the skillet, leaving the clams in the cans. Add the red pepper flakes. Bring to a simmer and cook until the liquid is reduced to ¾ cup, about 15 minutes.
4. Add the clams to the broth and cook until heated through, about 1 minute. Turn off the heat and let sit for 1 minute.

5. Add the butter, stirring in each cube until fully melted before adding the next one. Stir in the lemon zest. Add zucchini noodles and toss to coat.

6. To serve, divide between four plates or shallow bowls. Top with parsley and black pepper, and serve with lemon wedges, if desired.

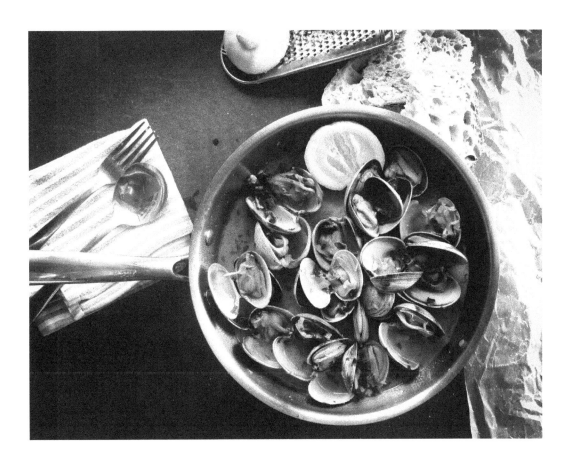

Nutrition:

Calories: 267

Carbs: 44.1g

Fat: 6.8g

Fiber: 7.2g

Protein: 7.3g

45. Chicken Mushroom Shrimp Mix with Green Onions

Preparation time: 10 minutes

Cooking time: 20 minutes

Servings: 4

Ingredients:

- 1/2 pound mushrooms, roughly sliced off
- Table salt and black pepper to the taste
- 1/4 mug mayonnaise
- 2 Tablespoon sriracha
- 1/2 tsp. paprika
- 1/4 tsp. xanthan gum
- 1 green onion stalk, sliced off
- 20 shrimp, raw, peeled and deveined
- 2 chicken breasts, boneless and skinless
- 2 handfuls spinach leaves
- 2 teaspoons lime juice
- 1 tablespoon coconut oil
- 1/2 tsp. red pepper, crushed
- 1 tsp. garlic grinding grains

Directions:

1. Warm up a dish with the oil over moderate gigantic warmth, embed chicken bosoms, season with table salt, pepper, red pepper and garlic pounding grains, plan for 8 minutes, flip and get ready for 6 minutes more.
2. Supplement mushrooms, more table salt and pepper and plan for a couple of moments.

3. Warm up another dish over moderate warmth, embed shrimp, sriracha, paprika, xanthan and mayo, shake and get ready until shrimp turn pink.
4. Eliminate heat, embed lime squeeze and shake everything.
5. Serve spinach on plates, appropriate chicken and mushroom, top with shrimp consolidate, decorate with green onions.

Nutrition:

Calories: 171

Carbs: 24g

Fat: 6.4g

Proteins: 6.2g

Chapter 8. Appendix Measurement Conversions

Volume Equivalents (Liquid)

US STANDARD	US STANDARD (OUNCES)	METRIC (APPROXIMATE)
2 tablespoons	1 fl. oz.	30 mL
1/4 cup	2 fl. oz.	60 mL
1/2 cup	4 fl. oz.	120 mL
1 cup	8 fl. oz.	240 mL
1 1/2 cups	12 fl. oz.	355 mL
2 cups or 1 pint	16 fl. oz.	475 mL
4 cups or 1 quart	32 fl. oz.	1 L
1 gallon	128 fl. oz.	4 L

Volume Equivalents (Dry)

US STANDARD	METRIC (APPROXIMATE)
1/8 teaspoon	0.5 mL
1/4 teaspoon	1 mL
1/2 teaspoon	2 mL
3/4 teaspoon	4 mL
1 teaspoon	5 mL
1 tablespoon	15 mL
1/4 cup	59 mL
1/3 cup	79 mL

1/2 cup	118 mL
2/3 cup	156 mL
3/4 cup	177 mL
1 cup	235 mL
2 cups or 1 pint	475 mL
3 cups	700 mL
4 cups or 1 quart	1 L

Oven Temperatures

FAHRENHEIT	CELSIUS (APPROXIMATE)
250°F	120°C
300°F	150°C
325°F	165°C
350°F	180°C
375°F	190°C
400°F	200°C
425°F	220°C
450°F	230°C

Conclusion

The Pegan diet is designed to be flexible, allowing you to adjust the type of foods you eat according to your needs. You can follow the diet as is, or you can modify it to fit your individual needs and preferences. As a basis, this regimen emphasizes eating foods that are higher in protein and low in carbohydrates. It also discourages eating meals that contain meat, dairy, processed foods, and refined sugar.

This popular weight loss program involves eating healthy foods in an easy-to-follow way. With this diet plan, you can lose weight and maintain your new healthy lifestyle all while eating tasty foods. What many people don't realize is that there are many benefits to the diet besides just losing weight. For example, it is also a simple way to manage your nutrition since it guarantees that you will get all the nutrients you need to grow and stay fit.

The Pegan diet has been used with success by people for over ten years. Over time, the Pegan diet has become one of the most popular diet plans in the world. Nowadays, it is used by many people across America and other parts of the world.

CPSIA information can be obtained
at www.ICGtesting.com
Printed in the USA
BVHW051249230621
610212BV00014B/1999